Mayo Clinic on
Hearing and Balance

MAYO
CLINIC | Mayo Clinic Press

MAYO CLINIC

Medical Editor Jamie M. Bogle, Au.D., Ph.D.

Publisher Daniel J. Harke

Editor in Chief Nina E. Wiener

Managing Editor Stephanie K. Vaughan

Art Director Stewart J. Koski

Production Design Darren L. Wendt

Illustration and Photography Mayo Clinic Media Support Services, Mayo Clinic Medical Illustration and Animation

Editorial Research Librarians Abbie Y. Brown, Edward (Eddy) S. Morrow Jr., Erika A. Riggin, Katherine (Katie) J. Warner

Copy Editors Miranda M. Attlesey, Donna L. Hanson, Nancy J. Jacoby, Julie M. Maas

Indexer Carol Roberts

Contributors Aleta K. Capelle; Michael J. Cevette, Ph.D.; Nicholas L. Deep, M.D.; Omolola O. Famuyide, P.T., D.P.T.; Adam M. Goulson, Au.D.; Cynthia A. Hogan, Ph.D.; Sarah (Sarah Oakley) O. Holbert, C.C.C.-A; Elaine D. Johnson-Siekmann, P.T., D.P.T.; Brian H. Kaihoi; Jon R. (Joey) Keillor; Amanda J. Knapp; Heather L. LaBruna; Giau N. Le, Au.D., C.C.C.-A.; Devin L. McCaslin, Ph.D.; Gayla L. Poling, Ph.D.; Manami H. Shah; Helga I. Smars, P.T.; Greta C. Stamper, Au.D., Ph.D.; Peter A. Weisskopf, M.D.; David A. Zapala, Ph.D.

We acknowledge with gratitude the individuals and families who shared their experiences with hearing loss and balance issues in this book: Teresa Bowers; Judith Collins; Lexi Grafe; Ken Larson; Matt, Melinda, and Aida Little; Scott Malmstrom; Julie Metternich Olson; Sue Sherek; Joyce Sherman; and Greta Stamper. Additional gratitude goes to Matthew L. Carlson, M.D.; Colin L. W. Driscoll, M.D.; Lori E. Hubka; Terra M. Paulson; and Colleen D. Young for their support in developing the personal stories in this book.

Published by Mayo Clinic Press

© 2022 Mayo Foundation for Medical Education and Research (MFMER)

For bulk sales to employers, member groups and health-related companies, contact Mayo Clinic, 200 First St. SW, Rochester, MN 55905, or send an email to SpecialSalesMayoBooks@mayo.edu.

ISBN 978-1-893005-72-3

Library of Congress Control Number: 2021942614

Printed in the United States of America

Some images within this content were created prior to the COVID-19 pandemic and do not demonstrate proper pandemic protocols. Please follow all recommended CDC guidelines for masking and social distancing.

Table of Contents

Preface

Hearing allows you to have meaningful conversations and experience the world around you. A solid sense of balance helps you feel steady and confident when you move. When they're in good working order, your ears provide what you need for both hearing and balance.

Problems with your ears, whether they're related to hearing, balance or both, can chip away at your self-confidence, affect how well you communicate, and make life less enjoyable overall.

If you're having trouble hearing, you may feel uncomfortable in social situations. You may feel frustrated as you try to go about your day. You may find it easier to withdraw from others. People may see you as timid or disconnected and give up trying to communicate with you.

Likewise, dizziness and balance issues can cause their own variety of struggles. When you're walking, transitioning from a sidewalk to grass may be difficult. It may be hard to get out of bed in the middle of the night without stumbling. Dizziness and balance problems can make it more likely that you'll fall and get seriously injured, and your fear of falling may keep you from leaving your home to interact with others. Issues with balance and dizziness can have a number of different causes, and problems with the ears are among them.

In the chapters that follow, you'll learn how your ears are connected to hearing loss and balance disorders. You'll also learn what role you can play in living well with and even preventing hearing loss and balance disorders.

Jamie M. Bogle, Au.D., Ph.D.

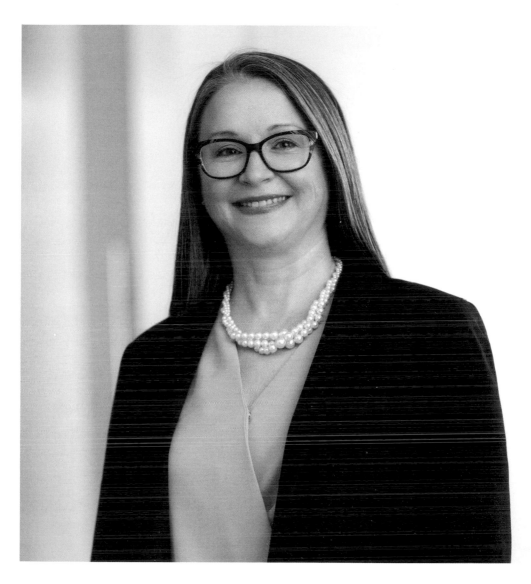

Jamie M. Bogle, Au.D., Ph.D., is a Mayo Clinic audiologist who specializes in evaluating children and adults with dizziness and imbalance issues. She is the chair of the Division of Audiology in the Department of Otolaryngology (ENT)/Head and Neck Surgery at Mayo Clinic in Scottsdale and Phoenix, Ariz., and an assistant professor of audiology at the Mayo Clinic College of Medicine and Science. Dr. Bogle also serves as associate editor for the *American Journal of Audiology* and has authored numerous scientific papers and addressed many hearing- and balance-related topics as an instructor and guest lecturer.

ARE YOU EXPERIENCING HEARING LOSS?

The following questions are based on guidance from the National Institute on Deafness and Other Communication Disorders. These questions can help you decide whether to make an appointment with your doctor or a hearing specialist.

- ☐ Do you have trouble hearing on the telephone?
- ☐ Do you have to strain to understand conversations?
- ☐ Do you have trouble following a conversation when two or more people are talking at the same time?
- ☐ Do you have trouble hearing in a situation with a noisy background?
- ☐ Do people say that you turn the TV volume up too high?
- ☐ Do you find yourself asking people to repeat themselves?
- ☐ Do many people you talk to seem to mumble or not speak clearly?
- ☐ Do people get annoyed because you misunderstand what they say?
- ☐ Do you respond inappropriately to what people say?
- ☐ Do you have trouble understanding people who have high-pitched voices or are soft-spoken — often women and children?

If you answered yes to three or more of these questions, ask someone who knows you well to consider these questions with you in mind. He or she might notice signs of hearing loss in you long before you do and prompt you to get help. From there, consider asking your doctor about having a hearing evaluation.

ARE YOU EXPERIENCING IMBALANCE OR DIZZINESS?

The following questions are based on guidance from the National Institute on Deafness and Other Communication Disorders. These questions can help you decide whether to make an appointment with your doctor or a balance specialist.

☐ Do you feel unsteady?
☐ Do you feel like the room is spinning around you, even for a moment?
☐ Do you feel like you're moving when you're sitting still?
☐ Have you lost your balance or fallen?
☐ Do you feel like you're falling?
☐ Do you feel lightheaded or as if you might faint?
☐ Is your vision blurry?
☐ Do you feel disoriented or lose your sense of location?

If you answered yes to any of these questions, talk to your doctor.

PART 1

Hearing and balance: Why do they matter?

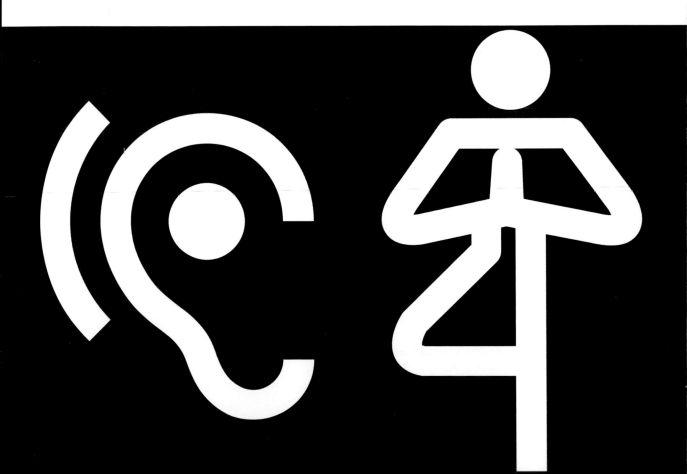

1

Common issues, one link

If you have hearing loss, you're not alone. Hearing loss affects about 36 million people in the United States and becomes more common with age. About 1 in 3 Americans between ages 65 and 74 has hearing loss. This number jumps to 1 in 2 in adults over age 75.

Worldwide, around 466 million people have severe hearing loss. That number is expected to jump to over 900 million by 2050. This number would be much higher if it included cases of mild hearing loss.

Although hearing loss generally becomes more common with age, it can occur at any age due to factors like noise exposure, trauma, genetics and illness.

Balance and dizziness, like hearing loss, affect many people. According to some estimates, more than a third of adults age 40 and older in the U.S. have experienced issues with dizziness or balance. About 8 million American adults say they have an ongoing problem with balance, and 2½ million adults in the U.S. have chronic

LEARN MORE

Colin L. W. Driscoll, M.D., chair, Department of Clinical Genomics, Mayo Clinic, talks about the health consequences of untreated hearing loss: links.mayoclinic.org/untreatedloss issues with dizziness. Among adults over age 65, almost a third experience dizziness to some extent.

Dizziness is a common reason adults visit their doctors. In fact, more than 10 million people in the U.S. see a doctor for dizziness issues each year. Dizziness is more common among older adults, but anyone of any age can experience it.

Dizziness can increase the risk of a fall and may cause you to fear doing even the most common everyday tasks. This fear can lead to a downward spiral: You feel less confident doing ordinary tasks, so you stop doing them. In turn, you sit more and become inactive. This leads to weak and less flexible muscles, stiff joints, fatigue, frustration and even depression.

While hearing and balance disorders are separate and distinct issues, they often have something in common: your ears.

The ears are amazing acoustic devices, unmatched by human ingenuity or invention. In a person with typical hearing, the ears — in combination with the brain — can almost instantly turn sound waves from the external world into the recognizable voice of a loved one, the call of a songbird or a crack of thunder. Just as some parts of the inner ear make it so you can hear, intricate parts of your inner ear work in concert to ensure that you move safely about your day.

Here's a closer look at the important structures that make up the ear and how they work to help you hear and stay balanced.

PARTS OF THE EAR

You likely already know what your ear looks like, with its recognizable flap of cartilage on each side of your head. But

WHAT DOES DIZZINESS FEEL LIKE?

If you're not sure how to describe what dizziness feels like to you, here are some possible descriptions you may use. You may say you feel:

- Like the room is spinning
- Like you're spinning in a room, even though you're not moving
- Lightheaded
- Faint
- Unsteady
- Like you might pass out
- Like you're going to lose your balance
- Like you're floating
- Woozy
- Like your head is heavy

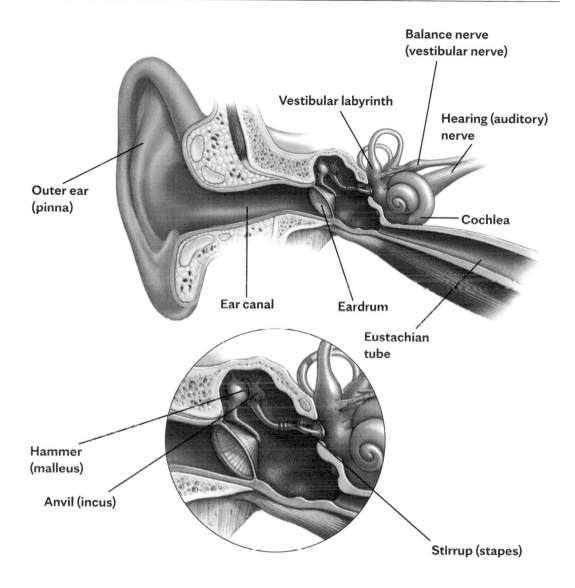

Balance nerve
(vestibular nerve)

Vestibular labyrinth

Hearing (auditory)
nerve

Outer ear
(pinna)

Cochlea

Ear canal

Eardrum

Eustachian
tube

Hammer
(malleus)

Anvil (incus)

Stirrup (stapes)

Middle ear

there's much more to your ears than what you see every day. Three complex, interconnected sections of the ear are used for hearing and balance. They're known as the outer ear, middle ear and inner ear.

Here's more on each part of the ear and how it relates to hearing and balance. See where all of these parts are located in the illustration below and on page 15.

Outer ear

The outer ear is what sticks out from each side of the head. It's made up of folds of skin and cartilage, called the pinna and

EAR ANATOMY

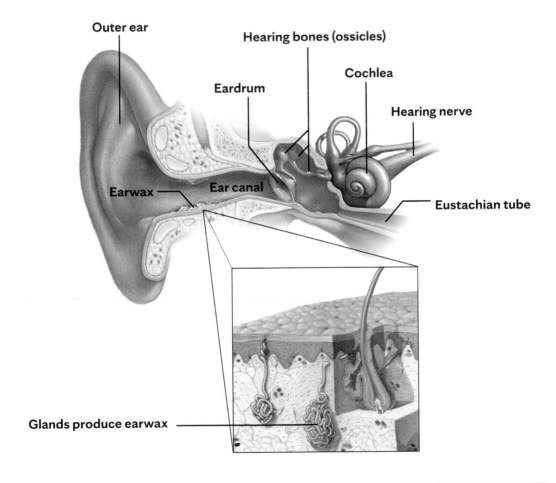

Outer ear

Hearing bones (ossicles)

Cochlea

Eardrum

Hearing nerve

Earwax

Ear canal

Eustachian tube

Glands produce earwax

the ear canal. The ear canal is an inch-long passageway that leads to the eardrum. The eardrum is a thin, taut membrane at the end of the ear canal. The eardrum separates the outer ear from the middle ear.

The skin lining the ear canal contains tiny hairs and glands that produce earwax, or cerumen (suh-ROO-mun). The hairs and earwax serve as cleaning mechanisms for the ear canal. They repel water, protect against bacteria, and keep foreign objects like dirt from slipping through the ear canal and reaching the eardrum.

How it helps you hear

The cupped shape of the outer ear (pinna) gathers sound waves from the environment around you. From there, the outer ear directs sound waves toward the ear canal. When they arrive in the ear canal, sound waves cause the eardrum to vibrate. See how this works below.

HOW HEARING WORKS

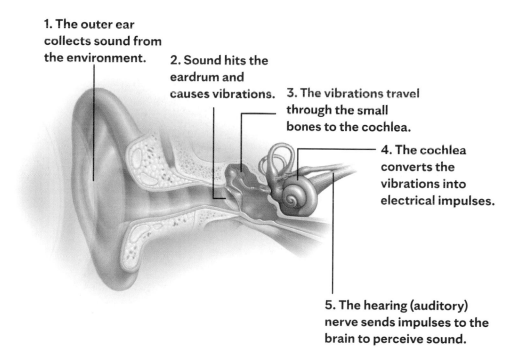

1. The outer ear collects sound from the environment.

2. Sound hits the eardrum and causes vibrations.

3. The vibrations travel through the small bones to the cochlea.

4. The cochlea converts the vibrations into electrical impulses.

5. The hearing (auditory) nerve sends impulses to the brain to perceive sound.

Middle ear

The middle ear is an air-filled cavity behind the eardrum. Lodged in the temporal bone of the skull, it houses three tiny bones called ossicles.

The ossicles (OS-ih-kuls) have scientific names, but each is known by a name that best describes its shape: the hammer (malleus), anvil (incus) and stirrup (stapes). Together, the ossicles form a bridge between the eardrum and the membrane-covered entrance to the inner ear.

A narrow channel called the eustachian (u-STAY-shun) tube connects the middle ear to the back of the nose and upper part of the throat — an area called the naso-pharynx (nay-zoh-FAR-inks).

The eustachian tube usually remains closed until you swallow or yawn. Then it opens briefly to equalize the air pressure within the middle ear to the air pressure that's outside — you may feel and hear a pop when this occurs. Maintaining equal air pressure on both sides of the eardrum allows the membrane to vibrate easily.

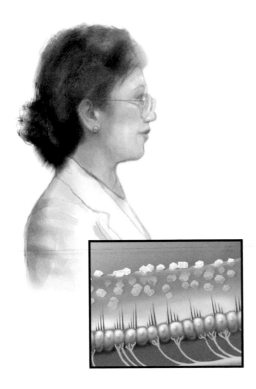

When the head is upright, the tiny hair cells of the vestibular system also are upright.

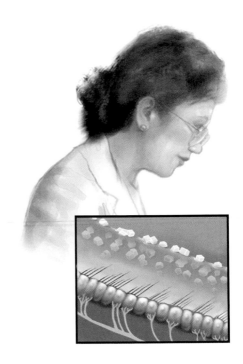

When the head tilts forward, gravity sensors pull the hair cells forward and tell the brain that the head is tipped forward.

How it helps you hear

Sound waves are transmitted through the ossicles. Each bone moves back and forth, much like a small lever, to increase the sound level that reaches the inner ear. A tiny muscle is attached to the hammer on one end of the ossicular bridge, and another tiny muscle to the stirrup at the other end.

Inner ear

The inner ear contains the most sophisticated part of the hearing mechanism: the fluid-filled, snail-shaped cochlea (KOK lee-uh). The inner ear also contains a structure called the vestibular labyrinth, which assists with your sense of balance.

How it helps you hear

The cochlea translates incoming sound waves into signals that can be understood by the brain. Tiny sensors (hair cells) in the cochlea receive sound waves, amplify them and turn them into electrical impulses that are then sent to the brain along the hearing (auditory) nerve.

How it helps with balance

The vestibular labyrinth is located just behind the cochlea and consists of three fluid-filled loops (semicircular canals) and two gravity sensors. These sensors contain hair cells that are sensitive to movement. These organs track every motion of your body, helping keep you

aware of turning motions and where your head is in relation to the ground. See how the gravity sensors work in the image on page 18.

Anytime you move in any direction, the fluid in your vestibular labyrinth stimulates hair cells that tell your brain about your movements. In turn, your brain responds to these messages, telling the rest of your body how to respond so that you stay balanced. For example, your brain may tell your eyes to stay focused in a certain direction or tell your muscles that they need to respond quickly. Later in this book, you'll learn more about the vestibular labyrinth and its link to symptoms like dizziness and vertigo.

Now you have a basic idea of how the ears are connected to hearing and balance. The next chapter details the everyday choices you can make to nurture both.

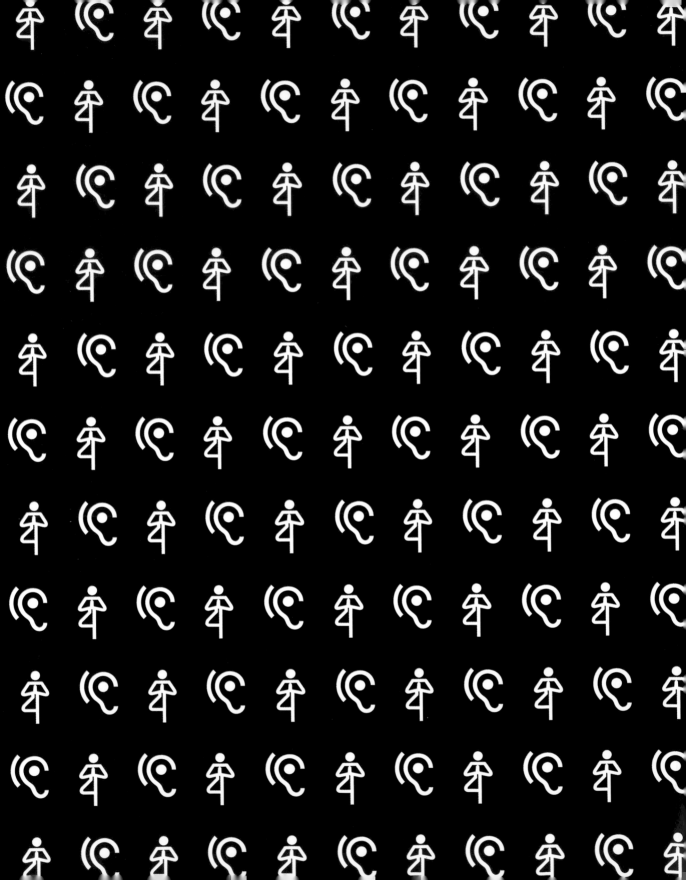

2

Hearing, balance and overall health

While your ears provide the tools you need for hearing and balance, your ears don't act alone. Many facets of your overall health and wellness also play a role. Your everyday choices make a difference in how well you hear and stay balanced.

In this chapter, you'll learn about some of the everyday habits that matter most.

FOLLOW A HEALTHY DIET

You're likely already familiar with the basics of a healthy diet. Making nutritious choices and limiting less healthy foods and beverages are key.

Here's more on the ways nutrition can help support your hearing and balance.

How it helps you hear

Researchers have found that a healthy diet can help protect against hearing loss in many ways.

For one, a healthy diet helps lower blood pressure and cholesterol, which keeps blood moving smoothly through your body. This means that blood flows well to the cochlea, the part of the ear that translates sound waves into signals your brain can understand. Good nutrition can also keep your brain working well and protect the nerve pathways between your ears and your brain.

A low-calorie diet that limits salt, saturated fat and sugar can make it less likely that you'll experience hearing loss. The more vegetables and fruits, the better.

How it helps with balance

Similar dietary habits help with balance. Limiting salt, for example, is often recommended as a treatment for balance disorders like Ménière's disease. A low-salt diet can help prevent dizziness episodes. Likewise, getting plenty of fresh vegetables and fruits and limiting processed foods help control salt and sugar intake. Experts also suggest drinking plenty of fluids and evenly spacing meals and amounts of food throughout the day.

These choices help regulate the fluid in the inner ear that helps with balance.

What you can do

Many hearing and balance experts recommend the Dietary Approaches to Stop Hypertension (DASH) diet, which focuses on reducing the sodium in the diet and eating foods rich in nutrients that help lower blood pressure, like potassium, calcium and magnesium.

BE GOOD TO YOUR HEART

Your heart pumps blood throughout your body. It ensures that there's enough blood for all of the processes of daily life, including your hearing and balance.

How it helps you hear

Although heart disease may not directly cause hearing loss, the two are related. When it's damaged, the heart can't pump enough blood for the ears to function. Without enough blood, the structures in the ear become damaged. This leads to permanent hearing loss.

Likewise, the network of blood vessels throughout your body needs to be robust enough to get blood from the heart to your ears and brain so you can hear. Healthy arteries are flexible and elastic, but over time, they can harden. This condition is known as arteriosclerosis. Another blood vessel issue, called atherosclerosis, happens when fats, cholesterol and other substances collect in your arteries and on your artery walls. The resulting plaques restrict blood flow. By reducing the blood supply to your ears and brain, these heart-related conditions can increase your risk of hearing loss.

Earlier, you learned how tiny sensors (hair cells) in the cochlea receive sound waves and send them on to your brain. These sensors rely on a steady supply of oxygen from your heart and blood vessels. When your hair cells don't get the oxygen they need, they die — and they can't be replaced. Once they're gone, they're lost forever. This is yet another example of how a strong heart and system of blood vessels keeps blood pumping to your ears and brain so that all hearing-related processes work well.

How it helps with balance

For similar reasons, the health of your heart and blood vessels is also critical to balance. Just as hair cells in your cochlea are necessary for hearing, hair cells in the

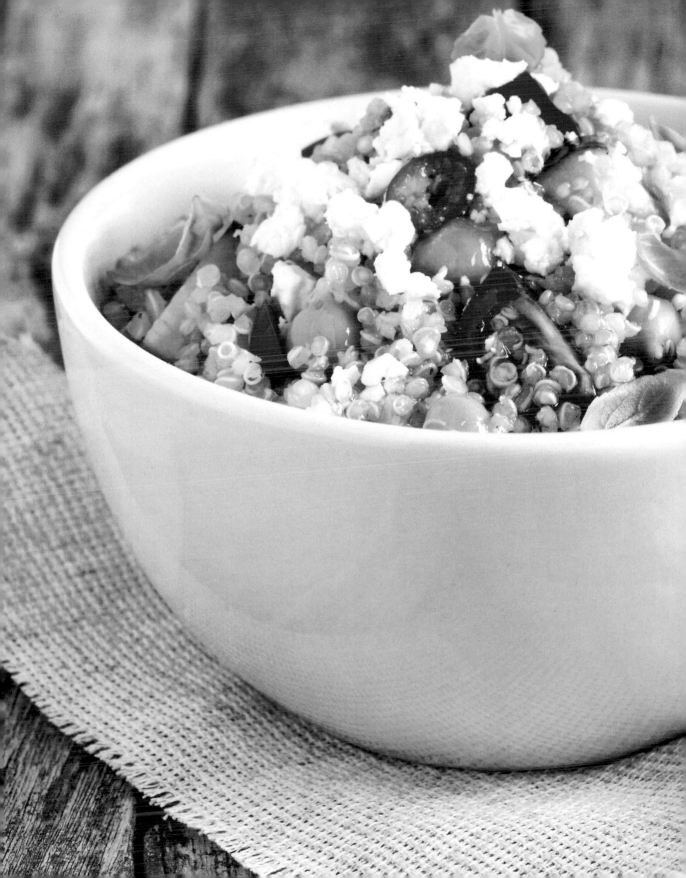

vestibular labyrinth keep tabs on the fluid in your ears. In turn, this sensitive system helps you keep your balance.

Just as with hair cells for hearing, you can't get hair cells for balance back once you lose them. But a properly functioning heart and system of blood vessels can help keep your hair cells healthy by giving them the oxygen-rich blood they need.

What you can do

Exercise that gets your lungs and heart pumping is one of the best ways to keep your heart and blood vessels strong. Aim for at least 30 to 60 minutes of activity a day. Regular, daily physical activity can lower your risk of heart disease and make it less likely that you'll develop other conditions that may put a strain on your heart, like high blood pressure, high cholesterol and type 2 diabetes.

If you haven't been active for a while, slowly work your way up to this goal. Even short bouts of activity offer benefits.

MANAGE OR PREVENT DIABETES

Like heart disease, type 2 diabetes can cause problems with blood vessels in the

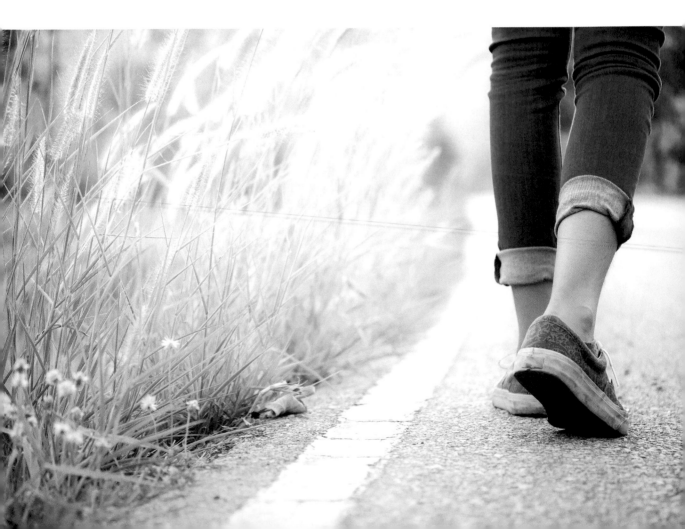

ears. These effects can contribute to hearing loss and balance challenges. Type 2 diabetes can also affect hearing and balance in other ways.

Here's more on the effects of type 2 diabetes on hearing and balance.

How it affects hearing

Over time, high blood sugar damages the small blood vessels and nerves in the inner ear that enable you to hear. This makes it harder for enough blood to get to the ears and the brain. In addition, high blood sugar can damage the nerve pathways that get sound waves from the ears to the brain.

According to some estimates, hearing loss is twice as common in people who have diabetes as it is in people who don't. Even people with prediabetes — blood sugar that's higher than usual but not high enough to be considered type 2 diabetes — are more likely to have hearing loss.

How it affects balance

As with hearing, high blood sugar causes issues with balance because it damages the small blood vessels and nerves in the inner ear. Type 2 diabetes can also affect the fluids in your inner ear that help you stay balanced.

But type 2 diabetes is linked to dizziness and balance issues for other reasons as well. For example, it can damage your vision, and it can affect your sense of self-movement and body position. It can also damage the nerves that give feeling to your feet. This is why unsteadiness and falls are common in people with type 2 diabetes. Changes in blood sugar level also can cause dizziness.

What you can do

Whether you have type 2 diabetes or not, there are steps you can take to manage your blood sugar level and prevent these effects. When it comes to your diet, count carbs. Eat balanced meals regularly. And avoid sugar-sweetened beverages. Exercise helps, too. Physical activity helps your body use insulin efficiently, and at the same time, your muscles are using sugar for energy. Managing stress is another way to keep blood sugar in check. When you're stressed, your body produces hormones that can cause your blood sugar level to rise. And when you're feeling stressed, it may be harder for you to stick to healthy habits like eating well and exercising.

Diet, exercise and stress management are three ways to keep your blood sugar from spiking to levels that can damage your hearing and balance.

MOVE YOUR BODY

You just learned that physical activity can help prevent diabetes-related damage that can affect hearing and balance. But exercise also offers many other protective benefits.

How it affects hearing

As people age, many become less active for a variety of reasons. In turn, less physical activity has been linked to hearing loss in older adults. The good news is that the reverse is also true: If you stay active as you age, your risk of hearing loss decreases.

In part, researchers think physical activity keeps a steady supply of oxygen flowing to the delicate structures of the ear involved in hearing. Experts also suspect that exercise is helpful because of its role in managing body weight. Evidence suggests that maintaining a healthy weight can make hearing loss less likely.

How it affects balance

Regular movement improves balance and reduces the risk of falls. Specific balance exercises can help you maintain your balance — and your confidence — at any age. Tai chi, dance, yoga, and postural awareness, strengthening and resistance, and water exercises are all examples.

Nearly any activity that keeps you on your feet and moving — even walking — can help you maintain good balance. Balance training can be done anywhere, anytime. You'll find balance exercises to practice later in this book.

What you can do

Get regular physical activity. Do activities you enjoy; they're the ones you'll most likely stick with over time. Remember: All activity counts!

TAKE CARE OF YOUR BONES

Strong bones are critical to both hearing and balance. Here's why.

How they affect hearing

Your inner ear, your hearing organ, is housed in the temporal bone. Your temporal bone protects your inner ear. Any bone loss in the temporal bone may lead to damage in the inner ear that causes hearing impairment. Bone loss can also damage the tiny bones within your inner ear. Without these bones, sound waves can't get to your brain.

Osteoporosis can lead to hearing loss in indirect ways as well. For example, the risk of heart attack and stroke is higher in people with osteoporosis. Heart attack and stroke can damage blood vessels, making it more difficult for blood to get to your ears and your brain. Good blood flow is necessary for all of the processes involved in hearing.

In addition, reduced bone density may alter the chemical processes your inner ear needs to function.

How they affect balance

Like your hearing organ, your balance system is housed in the temporal bone. As with hearing, osteoporosis can affect balance by causing a loss of density in the temporal bone. Likewise, bone loss can alter how your inner ear functions. All of these changes affect how well your balance system operates.

Osteoporosis also makes benign paroxysmal positional vertigo (BPPV) more likely. BPPV, which you'll read about in Chapter 15, is one of the most common causes of vertigo, the sudden feeling that you're spinning or that the inside of your head is spinning.

And while osteoporosis can damage bones and lead to problems with balance, it also seems that the opposite is true, that problems with balance may play a role in the development of osteoporosis. That's because your balance system works with your nervous system to keep a cycle of bone growth in motion. Together, these two systems are responsible for maintaining healthy bones.

What you can do

Experts don't know yet if early detection and treatment of osteoporosis can reduce the risk of hearing loss and balance issues, but it may. Plus, taking care of your bones has been shown to be important for a host of reasons, including reducing your risk of an injury-causing fall.

Following a diet that includes sources of healthy protein and calcium, maintaining a healthy weight, and getting enough calcium and vitamin D are all helpful. When you exercise, combine strength

training with weight-bearing exercises like walking and balance exercises like those featured later in this book.

The stage is set. You now have a foundational idea of how the ears work and how your daily choices can affect your hearing and balance. In the next several chapters, you'll learn about different types of hearing loss and balance disorders, what causes them, how they're treated, and how you can live well with them — and possibly prevent them.

Common hearing and balance issues

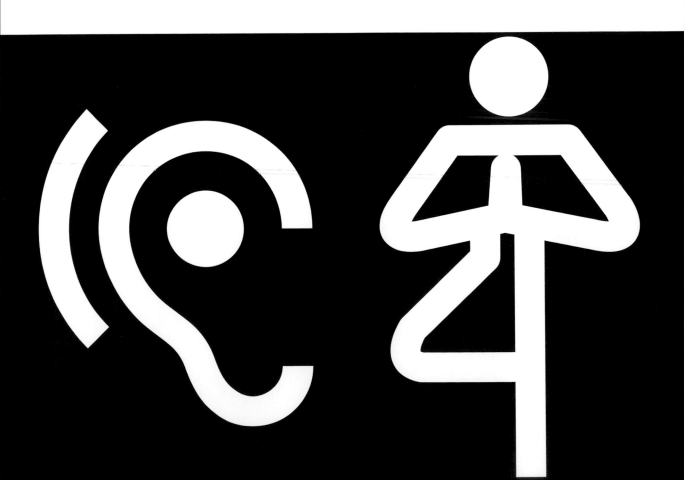

PART 2

CHAPTER

3

Concerns with the outer ear and middle ear

Working together, the outer ear and the middle ear make sure sound waves get to the inner ear. This allows strong, clear signals to get to the brain, where they're turned into sounds that you recognize.

When something keeps sound waves from passing through the outer ear and middle ear, you have conductive hearing loss. Often, the inner ear functions as it usually would.

When you have conductive hearing loss, all of the sounds you hear seem muffled. Sounds that are soft or faint to someone with typical hearing become inaudible.

A number of problems can keep sound waves from getting to the inner ear. Common causes of conductive hearing loss include too much earwax, ruptured

eardrum or infection that causes a fluid buildup in the middle ear. Other causes include cysts and benign tumors.

Conductive hearing loss can often be reversed with treatment. Sometimes, simple self-care is enough. Other times, you may need medication or surgery. Another piece of good news: Problems with the outer ear and middle ear generally don't cause permanent damage.

In this chapter, you'll learn about many of the common causes of conductive hearing loss and how they're treated.

OUTER EAR PROBLEMS

More often than not, problems with the outer ear aren't serious. But they can be uncomfortable and annoying. An outer ear infection, for example, can cause ear pain or itching, a swollen ear canal, and drainage of pus. Pus that blocks the ear canal can cause temporary hearing loss.

Self-care and treatment from a doctor when necessary are usually enough to resolve outer ear problems and restore hearing. Here's more on the most common causes of outer ear problems.

Earwax blockage

The skin that lines the outer part of your ear canal has glands that produce a waxy substance. Commonly known as earwax, you may hear it described by its medical name, cerumen. This wax is a natural defense. Its oils help keep the skin of the ear canal soft and protect the skin from water. It traps dust and other foreign particles that collect in the outer ear, keeping them from injuring your eardrum (tympanic membrane). Earwax also helps keep bacteria from growing.

Usually, the skin in your ear canal grows in a pattern much like a conveyor belt. This carries earwax to the outer edge of the ear canal. Earwax is also wiped away when you clean your outer ear. But sometimes, you may produce more wax than your ear can remove. This causes wax to build up in your ear canal.

Generally, having too much earwax doesn't lead to hearing loss because it doesn't completely block the passageway. But many people clean their ears by inserting objects like cotton swabs,

hairpins, keys and fingers into the ear canal. These actions push the earwax farther into the passageway and impact it. Impacted earwax, as it builds, can reduce hearing by blocking sound vibrations in the ear canal.

An earwax blockage can make the ear feel full or plugged. Rarely, it can cause noise such as ringing, buzzing or roaring in the ears (tinnitus).

Treating earwax blockage

To remove excess earwax, self-care may be all you need. Take these steps:
- Soften the earwax with a few drops of baby oil, mineral oil or olive oil from an eyedropper twice a day for several days.
- When the earwax is softened, fill a bowl with water heated to body temperature. If the water is colder or hotter than your body temperature, you may feel dizzy when you follow the next few steps.
- With your head upright, grasp the top of your ear and pull upward. With your other hand, squirt water gently into your ear canal with a 3-ounce rubber-bulb syringe. Lower your head to the side and allow the water to drain into the bowl.
- You may need to repeat the previous step several times before the excess earwax falls out.
- Dry your ear carefully with a towel or hand-held hair dryer on low heat. Insert a few drops of an alcohol-vinegar preparation (half rubbing alcohol, half white vinegar) with an eyedropper to help dry your ear.

Earwax removers sold in stores (Debrox Earwax Removal Kit, Murine Ear Wax Removal System) can also help. One note of caution: Don't flush your ears without talking to your doctor first if you've ruptured an eardrum or had ear surgery. Flushing could lead to pain or infection.

What about ear candling? This involves placing a lit, hollow, cone-shaped candle into the ear to remove earwax. The idea is that the heat from the flame will create a vacuum seal and the earwax will stick to the candle. Research shows that this technique doesn't work and can cause injury, including burns. In addition, ear candling may actually push earwax deeper into the canal.

If you still have excess wax in your ears after trying self-care, talk to your doctor. Your doctor may repeat the steps you've taken or use special tools to remove the earwax.

Foreign object in the ear

An object like a piece of cotton from a swab, a bit of paper, an earplug or even an insect can get stuck in your ear. When this happens, you may notice a tickle in your ear. Your ear may also hurt or feel plugged.

Most foreign objects that lodge in the ear canal don't cause lasting hearing problems. But if an object is pushed too far into your ear, it may rupture your eardrum and damage your middle ear. In turn, this can lead to more-serious consequences.

Removing a foreign object

If an object gets lodged in your ear, don't stick anything in your ear to try to remove it. You may push the object farther into the ear, making it harder to remove and causing serious damage. Instead, try the following:

- Tilt your head toward the affected side and shake it gently toward the ground.
- If someone else can see the object, he or she may be able to gently remove it with tweezers.
- If you can't access the object, call your doctor or your local urgent care number. A doctor will need to remove the object with tiny forceps or suction or by flooding the ear with fluid. A doctor can also check for any damage to your ear.
- If an insect is lodged in your ear and it's still alive, tilt the affected ear upward. Insects instinctively crawl up, rather than down, to free themselves.
- If the insect doesn't exit the ear on its own, place a few drops of warm — not hot — baby oil, mineral oil or olive oil into the ear. Gently pull the top of your ear back and upward when you place the oil into your ear. Usually, this will help the insect float out.

Don't use oil to remove objects other than an insect. Also, don't apply oil if you have pain, bleeding or discharge from the ear. These can be signs and symptoms of a perforated eardrum.

Swimmer's ear

Swimmer's ear is an infection of the ear canal. Usually, it's caused by persistent moisture in the ear — like from frequent swimming — often in combination with a mild injury to the skin of the ear canal.

Scraping the ear canal to clean out earwax can cause the kind of mild injury that can contribute to swimmer's ear. The scraping action creates the ideal situation for bacteria and fungi to invade the ear canal and cause infection. Hairspray and hair dyes also may cause an infection or an allergic reaction that can lead to swimmer's ear. Swimmer's ear is most common in children and young adults.

Treating swimmer's ear

If your pain is mild and you don't have ear

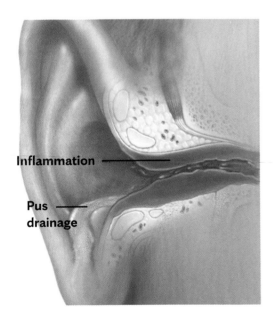

Inflammation

Pus drainage

With swimmer's ear, a small cut allows bacteria and fungi to invade the ear canal and cause an infection.

drainage or hearing loss, follow these self-care tips.

- Place a warm — not hot — heating pad over your ear. Don't lie on the heating pad.
- Consider taking ibuprofen (Advil, Motrin IB, others) or acetaminophen (Tylenol, others) to relieve pain.
- Keep water, fluids and other substances out of your ear canal while it's healing.
- Place a few drops of an alcohol-vinegar preparation (half rubbing alcohol, half white vinegar) in your ear after showering or swimming. The alcohol helps keep the skin of your ear canal dry, and the vinegar helps prevent bacterial and fungal growth from occurring. Do not do this if you have a known eardrum perforation.

If the pain doesn't go away after a day or two or if you have additional concerns, see your doctor. After cleaning your ear, your doctor may prescribe eardrops with a corticosteroid in them. These drops are used to relieve itching and decrease inflammation. Your doctor may also prescribe antibiotics to control infection. You may need to take oral antibiotics if you have a more-severe infection.

Swimmer's ear may lead to an infection of the bones and cartilage at the base of the skull. This type of infection is especially concerning for people with diabetes or a weakened immune system. This kind of infection is often accompanied by severe pain that gets worse over time. It can be life-threatening, and it usually requires long-term therapy with antibiotics therapy under the care of a team of specialists.

If you're a frequent swimmer, you may consider taking preventive measures like using over-the-counter drops (Auro-Dri, Swim-Ear, others) after you swim.

Surfer's ear

An overgrowth of bone can cause benign tumors to form in the ear canal. These tumors can get big enough that they block the ear canal and trap earwax and water. Ear infection also may develop.

This condition is known as surfer's ear because it develops in many people who surf. The growths are associated with long-term exposure to water and wind. The colder the water temperature, the higher the risk. That's because cold water surfers are more likely to develop these tumors than are warm-water surfers.

Treating surfer's ear

The tumors seen in surfer's ear grow slowly and often don't cause problems. If they block the ear canal, they can be removed with surgery. Surgery doesn't require a hospital stay, but recovery may take several weeks. The ear canal must be kept dry during recovery.

If a tumor causes an infection, antibiotics can take care of it.

Eardrum problems

The eardrum is a thin, elastic membrane. Its role is crucial: The eardrum is the gatekeeper for the sound waves traveling from your outer ear to your middle ear.

Although your eardrum is a resilient structure, it can experience infection or trauma that can keep your eardrum from working properly. As a result, sound waves may not be able to get to the middle ear. This can cause mild to moderate hearing loss that's usually temporary.

Here's more on common conditions that can affect the eardrum.

Infection and trauma

Ear infections cause fluid buildup in the middle ear that can put a lot of pressure on the eardrum. This pressure can force the eardrum to rupture. The pain caused by a fluid buildup usually improves once the eardrum has ruptured. That's because fluid draining out of the ear relieves the pressure. But chronic ear infections can gradually wear down the eardrum membrane and leave a hole.

The eardrum can also be ruptured by a sharp blow to the head or by a sudden increase in outside air pressure, such as from an explosion, slap across the ear or diving accident. The eardrum also can be punctured if you push an object, like a cotton swab or paper clip, too deeply into the ear canal.

Signs and symptoms of a ruptured eardrum include earache, partial hearing loss, noise like ringing, buzzing or roaring in the ears (tinnitus) and slight bleeding or discharge from the ear. In some cases, the three tiny bones (ossicles) in the middle ear may be damaged. This can cause more-severe hearing loss and, possibly, dizziness.

Often, a ruptured eardrum heals by itself without complications and with little or no permanent hearing loss. But some ruptures require medical help. If you think you've ruptured your eardrum, call your doctor right away. These self-care tips may help:

- Take aspirin or other pain relievers, if needed.
- Place a warm — not hot — heating pad over your ear.
- Keep your ear dry.
- Before showering, place a cotton ball coated with petroleum jelly into the ear canal to keep water out.

Your doctor may prescribe an antibiotic to make sure the infection is out of your

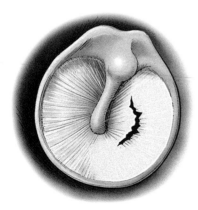

Although a ruptured eardrum usually will heal itself, there's still a risk of infection and hearing loss. It's important to see your doctor if you think your eardrum may be damaged.

ear and to help prevent it from recurring. He or she may also place a thin paper patch over your eardrum to seal the opening while it heals. If your eardrum hasn't healed within several months, you may need surgery.

Airplane ear

Airplane ear (ear barotrauma) is caused by a sharp difference between the air pressure in your middle ear and the outside pressure around you.

Usually, the narrow channel that connects the ear to the nose and upper throat (eustachian tube) lets air flow in and out of the middle ear. This air movement helps equalize pressure on both sides of the eardrum. You may notice clicks or popping sounds in your ears when you swallow or yawn to equalize the pressure.

Airplane ear occurs when you experience a sudden, drastic change in outside air pressure or water pressure. It may happen when you're making a rapid descent during an airplane landing or a deep-sea dive.

The rapid change in outside pressure restricts the airflow in the eustachian tube. In turn, the air pressure in the middle ear is less than the outside pressure. This imbalance causes the air-filled parts of the ear to compress and the eardrum to bow inward (retract).

The distortion of the eardrum interferes with the passage of sound waves, slightly reducing how well you hear. When you take part in activities that involve rapid changes in outside pressure, you may need to open your mouth or swallow frequently to equalize the pressure in your ears.

Signs and symptoms of airplane ear include pain in one or both ears, slight hearing loss, and a feeling that both ears are plugged.

An extreme pressure change or a completely blocked eustachian tube causes a more serious problem. Small blood vessels in your middle ear may rupture, filling your ear with blood and resulting in hearing loss.

Although airplane ear may cause discomfort, it usually doesn't cause permanent hearing loss. Pain usually goes away a few hours after the pressure has equalized and your hearing returns.

If you have to fly when you have a cold or nose congestion, try a nonprescription decongestant nasal spray (Afrin, Neo-Synephrine, others) 30 to 60 minutes before your flight. This helps keep your eustachian tubes clear. If you have a heart condition or blood pressure problems, talk to your doctor before taking a decongestant.

During the flight, chew gum or drink water to encourage swallowing. A method used by pilots is to pinch the nostrils shut, inhale and swallow, or to close the nostrils and try to blow air out the ears. The pop in your ears is a sign that air has gone through the eustachian tube to your middle ear.

If your symptoms don't go away, talk to your doctor. If your eustachian tube is blocked or can't work properly, you may need a small incision in your eardrum. The procedure used to do this is known as myringotomy (mir-ing-GOT-o-me). This helps equalize air pressure and allows fluid to be removed from your middle ear.

MIDDLE EAR PROBLEMS

Infections, cysts, tumors and irregular bone growths can affect your middle ear. These problems cause hearing loss when they disturb the eardrum or the tiny bones in the middle ear: the hammer (malleus), anvil (incus) and stirrup (stapes). Often, hearing can be restored with medicine or surgery. However, if a problem in the middle ear goes untreated and expands into the inner ear, you may lose hearing permanently.

Here are the main types of problems that can affect the middle ear.

Middle ear infection

A middle ear infection is often referred to as otitis media. It's associated with colds and other upper respiratory infections, which can block the eustachian tube. When the eustachian tube is blocked, the ear can't clear itself properly. This causes swelling and inflammation, and fluid builds up in the middle ear.

At the same time, bacteria from the nose, mouth or throat may travel through the lining of the eustachian tube and infect the trapped fluid in the middle ear. The infected fluid usually causes ear pain. It also causes a thick mucus or pus to form. Infected fluid may also keep the eardrum and ossicles from moving properly. This can cause hearing loss because sound waves can't move through the middle ear in the way that they need to.

Rarely, pressure from an infection may tear, or rupture, the eardrum. When this happens, the tear usually heals quickly, without lasting problems. An acute middle ear infection is a single, severe episode that starts fairly suddenly and usually lasts no more than two weeks.

Signs and symptoms of a middle ear infection include:
• Severe pain or pressure in the ear

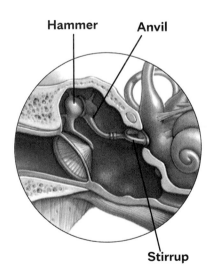

Middle ear problems can cause hearing loss when they disturb the eardrum or the tiny bones in the middle ear: the hammer (malleus), anvil (incus) and stirrup (stapes).

• Fever above 100 F
• Disrupted sleep
• Feeling like the ear is plugged

Other signs and symptoms may include dizziness, loss of balance, nausea, vomiting and drainage from the ear.

Although a middle ear infection may occur at any age, it's most common in young children. In fact, 5 out of 6 children will have at least one ear infection by their third birthday. This is partly due to the shape of a child's eustachian tube, which is shorter and more horizontal than an adult's is. When it's more horizontal in orientation, the eustachian tube is less likely to drain fluid well. In turn, the fluid may build up in the ear.

This trapped fluid is an ideal breeding ground for bacteria or viruses that cause infection. Sometimes, fluid remains trapped after the infection is gone. This can cause recurring infections, which you'll learn about later in this chapter.

How it's treated

The pain, fever or drainage of a middle ear infection is what will likely cause you to see a doctor. When your doctor looks in your ears, he or she may see that your eardrum is off-color, bulging or indented. You may have a test that measures your eardrum's movement (tympanometry). This test may show that your eardrum isn't moving well. Your doctor may also take a sample of the fluid draining from your ear to find out what's causing the infection.

Many ear infections heal on their own without treatment. With this in mind, you and your doctor may watch and wait before opting for antibiotics. If fluid in the ear isn't infected or if the infection is viral rather than bacterial, antibiotics won't help — and research shows that viruses cause most ear infections.

To ease ear pain, use over-the-counter pain relievers like ibuprofen (Advil, Motrin IB, others) or acetaminophen (Tylenol, others). While you wait for the medicine to take effect, try applying a cold pack or cold wet washcloth to the outer ear for 20 minutes. In place of a cold pack, you may use a warm compress.

Taking an antihistamine or decongestant may improve how you breathe through your nose. In turn, this may help increase airflow through the eustachian tube.

In follow-up visits, your doctor will likely check to see if the infection gets better or worse and watch for signs and symptoms of more-severe illness. Severe pain, high fever, pain behind the ear, trouble moving the muscles in your face, stiff neck, dehydration, difficulty breathing and extreme irritability are examples.

If your symptoms last more than 2 to 3 days, your doctor may prescribe an antibiotic. Unless your doctor knows what's causing your infection, you'll likely take an antibiotic that's effective against a range of bacteria. If the infection doesn't respond to one kind of antibiotic, your doctor may prescribe another one.

Once you start taking an antibiotic, it's important to take all of it, even if your symptoms improve. This ensures that all of the bacteria are killed.

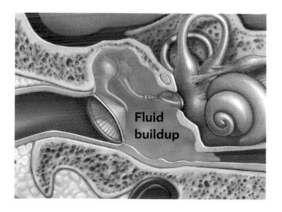 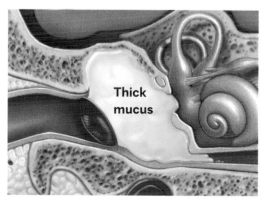

An ear infection (left) can happen when the eustachian tube gets blocked due to a cold or other respiratory infection. Fluid may build up in the middle ear where there's usually air. Bacteria from the nose and throat can infect the trapped fluid (right). This causes a thick mucus or pus to form. This is what keeps the eardrum and ossicles from moving as they usually do and causes hearing loss.

Fluid in the middle ear usually disappears 3 to 6 weeks after the infection clears up.

Chronic ear infection

Sometimes, you may have a low level of infection in your ear even after you've been treated for an ear infection. Other times, an infection leaves your ear at risk of future infections. Or ongoing swelling and irritation in the tissue behind your nasal passages may block the eustachian tube. These are just some of the ways that ear infections can become chronic, happening from time to time.

Chronic ear infections may seem milder than an acute infection. In fact, you may not even know you're experiencing a chronic infection until it's well established in your ear.

But a chronic ear infection can be more harmful than the acute type. A chronic ear infection can cause permanent ear damage and hearing loss.

When the eustachian tube is blocked often, middle ear tissue starts to thicken and get inflamed. Mucus trapped in the middle ear also thickens. The blocked tube can create a vacuum in the middle ear that, over time, can cause the eardrum to rupture or become deformed.

As these changes come about, the middle ear and inner ear structures start to break down. This causes permanent damage and hearing loss. Infection also can spread to the bone behind the ear (mastoid) — and even to the brain.

If pus is seeping from your ear canal, if your ear continually hurts, or if you experience hearing loss, seek medical attention. Your doctor can refer you to an audiologist, who can tell what kind of hearing loss you have and how severe it is.

Your doctor may also try to find the source of infection. A computerized tomography (CT) scan may be taken, albeit rarely, to check if infection has spread to the bone behind the ear.

ACUTE EAR INFECTION: KEY POINTS

- Urgent medical attention isn't usually needed for ear pain and possible ear infections.
- Most ear infections aren't serious and heal on their own without antibiotics.
- Pain relievers and other pain management strategies like warm or cold compresses are helpful for ear pain.
- Doctors most often recommend antibiotics for ear infections when ear pain lasts more than two or three days or if you have more-severe signs and symptoms.
- Seek immediate care if you start to have signs or symptoms of severe illness.

How it's treated

Medications and surgery are the two most common ways chronic ear infections are treated.

If nasal congestion from a cold or an allergy is contributing to your infection, your doctor may prescribe an antihistamine or a decongestant. This helps open the eustachian tube, helps you breathe better through your nose. It also helps air flow to and from the middle ear. However, some studies cast doubt on how well these drugs work with chronic ear infections.

Some doctors recommend taking low-dose antibiotics to keep middle ear infections from recurring. However, antibiotics haven't been shown to prevent these infections. Plus, widespread, prolonged use of antibiotics can contribute to the growth of drug-resistant bacteria.

If your middle ear is filled with fluid for more than three months and your eardrum isn't ruptured, you may need to have a small cut made in your eardrum to relieve pressure and help drain fluid. Hearing often improves right after this is done.

It usually takes less than 15 minutes to make the incision in the eardrum, suction out the fluid, and insert a metal or plastic tube into the hole. This tube stays in place to allow fluid to drain. Some tubes stay in place for up to a year and then fall out on their own. Others stay in longer and may need to be removed with surgery.

If your eardrum and ossicles have significant damage, you may need surgery to remove infected tissue and repair these structures. This procedure is known as tympanomastoidectomy (tim-puh-no-mas-toid-EK-tuh-me). The entire procedure may be done all at once. Or you may have surgery just to eliminate the infection first. Later on, surgery is performed to reconstruct the middle ear structures. Chronic ear infections often require more than one surgery.

Cholesteatoma

Cholesteatoma (koe-luh-ste-uh-TOE-muh) is a cyst commonly found in the middle ear or the bone behind the ear. It can occur when skin from the ear canal grows into the middle ear through a hole or tear in the eardrum. A blocked eustachian tube also can cause this cyst. The blockage creates a vacuum in the middle ear, bending your eardrum inward to form a pocket. Old skin cells get caught in the eardrum pocket and develop into a cystlike cholesteatoma.

Babies are sometimes born with this cyst when skin cells become trapped behind the eardrum.

Signs and symptoms of cholesteatoma include pus drainage from the ear, hearing loss, ear pain or fullness, dizziness, and weak muscles in the face.

A cholesteatoma isn't cancerous and won't spread. How much hearing loss it causes depends on how big the cyst is and where it's located. Often, this cyst will damage the delicate bones of the middle ear (ossicles) or make it hard for them to work. This causes significant hearing loss.

If it's not treated, this cyst may affect the cochlea and vestibular labyrinth of the inner ear, leading to permanent hearing loss and problems with balance. It can also damage the facial nerve. On rare occasions, it can cause an infection of the central nervous system (meningitis).

How it's treated

Surgery is needed to treat a cholesteatoma. If it's large or more invasive, you may need a series of operations to correct damage to the bones of your middle ear and possibly to rebuild them. If all of the cyst isn't removed, it will likely grow back, possibly requiring surgery later on. Although surgery generally doesn't require a hospital stay, some people need to stay overnight afterward.

In severe cases when a cholesteatoma is large or located in an area of the ear that's hard to access, you may have surgery to remove damaged parts of the bone behind your ear. This leaves a cavity that must be cleaned out from time to time, and it doesn't effectively restore lost hearing. Additional surgery may be needed to rebuild the ossicular chain in the middle ear if it's been damaged.

Other cysts and tumors

Less often, irregular growths may develop in the middle ear and tissues around it.

Most middle ear tumors aren't cancerous, but some are — and they can spread to other parts of the body. Tumors that aren't cancerous usually grow slowly. When they're cancerous, these tumors tend to grow more quickly.

If you have a tumor, it may feel like your ear is plugged. You may also have ringing, buzzing or roaring in your ears (tinnitus), hearing loss, drainage from the ear, dizziness, and loss of balance. You may also be unable to move the muscles in your face.

Talk to your doctor if you have any of these signs and symptoms. A CT scan or MRI scan can show if you have a tumor. If you do, your doctor may take a sample of it to see if it's cancerous.

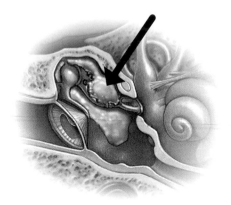

This cholesteatoma (see arrow) hasn't been treated. It has worn away the bones in the middle ear and ruptured the eardrum. When this cyst is removed with surgery, the eardrum may need to be patched, and the ossicles may need to be replaced with an artificial device.

The more common tumors are:

- **Glomus tympanicum and glomus jugulare.** These are masses of cells that make it hard for the three tiny bones of the middle ear (ossicles) to function. You'll recall that the ossicles move in a way that allows sound waves to get to the inner ear. A glomus tumor often causes a pulsing sound in the ear that accompanies each heartbeat. Most of these tumors aren't cancerous. However, on rare occasions, they can spread to the lymph nodes in the neck and become a more serious problem.
- **Squamous cell carcinoma.** Cancerous tumors of the ear are rare, but of those that occur, squamous cell carcinoma (SKWAY-mus sel car-sih-NO-muh) is the most common. This type of tumor develops in the skin cells of the outer ear and ear canal and spreads into the middle ear and the bony part behind the ear. Although sun and radiation exposure from tanning lamps and tanning beds can cause this type of skin cancer initially, this cancer can also develop on skin that's not exposed to sunlight, for reasons researchers don't yet understand. Ear pain, draining of fluid from the ear and long periods of bleeding from the ear are signs and symptoms of this type of cancer. If left untreated, this type of cancer is fatal.

How they're treated

Surgery and radiation may be used to treat tumors of the ear. Sometimes, especially in older adults, the tumors may simply be watched over time. With this approach, regular MRI or CT scans are taken to check the tumor for growth.

Surgery to remove a tumor is delicate and complex. It may involve removing some or all parts of the ear, depending on the nature and size of the tumor. This can result in permanent hearing loss. It can also cause a loss of function in the nerves leading to the face and throat, which can affect your voice and how well you can swallow.

It's important to treat a cancerous tumor right away. Radiation therapy may be used on its own or along with surgery. Radiation therapy is often used after surgery to destroy all remaining cancer cells.

Otosclerosis

Otosclerosis (o-toe-skluh-ROE-sis) develops when a growth of bone forms at the entrance to the inner ear (oval window). This growth causes the stirrup — one of the tiny bones in the middle ear — to get stuck to the oval window. In turn, the stirrup can no longer vibrate and help move sound waves to the inner ear.

For a small number of people with otosclerosis, hearing loss can be profound, especially if it affects the tissue in the cochlea of the inner ear. Other signs and symptoms of otosclerosis include dizziness, balance problems and tinnitus.

Otosclerosis is a frequent cause of conductive hearing loss in young adults. It's more common in women than in men and affects white people more often than individuals of other races. Signs and symptoms of the condition usually appear between the ages of 20 and 50. The disease develops over time and can affect one or both ears.

Research suggests that genetic makeup may make it more likely for someone to have this disease. Having one parent with the disorder generally makes someone 25% more likely to develop it. The risk doubles if both of parents have the disorder.

How it's treated

Because otosclerosis typically results in mild to moderate hearing loss and doesn't progress far beyond that, hearing aids or other hearing devices can help most people who have hearing loss caused by this condition.

Surgery is also an option. The fixed stirrup can be replaced with a tiny wire or another prosthesis. This procedure is known as a stapedotomy (stay-puh-DOT-uh-me). The prosthesis works as the stirrup did, allowing sound vibrations to pass from the eardrum to the inner ear. You may not notice improvement in your hearing until 3 to 6 weeks after surgery, but the improvement is usually permanent. In rare cases, though, this surgery may actually worsen hearing loss.

This surgery does pose possible drawbacks. The prosthesis may get displaced, a growth of bone may recur, or the part of the ear that the prosthesis is attached to may wear away. In rare cases, this surgery results in complete hearing loss in the affected ear or other complications, such as dizziness, ringing in the ear, taste disturbance or facial paralysis. If the disease gets worse after surgery, the prosthesis may not work as well over time.

If you have otosclerosis, you may be told to take tablets of sodium fluoride to help preserve hearing. But how well this works is under debate.

Advocates of this treatment say fluoride may help harden the bone growth, preventing changes in the inner ear and the hearing loss they may cause. However, fluoride is already present in most public water supplies in the U.S., so additional fluoride treatment is usually not needed.

Ossicular chain disruption

A traumatic head injury can cause the small bones of the middle ear (ossicles) to shift or break.

Trauma commonly causes problems where these bones connect, and often, one of the bones partially breaks. Fractures disrupt the chain of bones, causing a breakdown in the sound pathway from the eardrum to the inner ear. Significant hearing loss results.

How it's treated

Obviously, a complete medical examination is best following any serious head trauma. Tests can show what kind of hearing loss you have and how severe it is. If you still have hearing loss six months after the trauma, your doctor may suggest surgery or have you see an audiologist to discuss using a hearing aid.

If you have surgery, you'll likely have what's called ossiculoplasty (os-IH-coo-low-plas-tee). This attempts to rebuild the displaced ossicles or to replace them either with a prosthesis or with small pieces of bone or cartilage. Because the ossicles are tiny, this operation is delicate. You may not recover all of your hearing.

Although complications are rare, all types of ear surgery pose these risks:
• Total deafness in the affected ear
• Tinnitus
• Dizziness and loss of balance
• Damage to the facial nerve, resulting in changes to sense of taste or facial paralysis on the affected side

Your ear doctor will likely discuss such risks with you before any decision is made regarding surgery.

Sometimes, head trauma damages the cochlea, causing hearing loss in the inner ear that can't be repaired with surgery. In these cases, a hearing aid may be the best option.

Knowing how to spot the signs and symptoms of middle ear and outer ear issues can help with getting them treated quickly, before they have a chance to cause issues with hearing and balance.

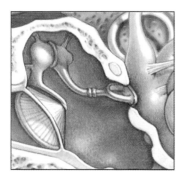 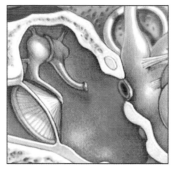 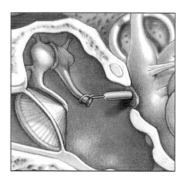

Surgery known as a stapedotomy is sometimes used to treat otosclerosis. With a stapedotomy, the stirrup that's stuck and no longer moving is partly or completely removed. It's then replaced with a tiny wire or another prosthesis that guides sound waves to the inner ear.

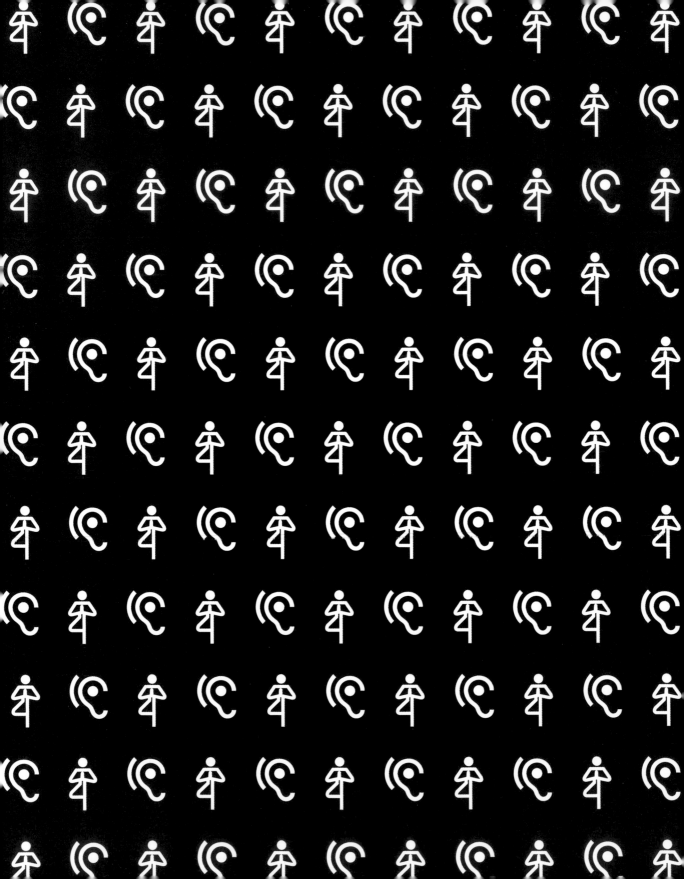

Problems of the inner ear

The inner ear is a critical way station that makes hearing and balance possible. The cells in the inner ear turn sound into a signal that the brain can understand. Fine hair cells and fluid in the inner ear help with balance.

So when the inner ear fails to work properly, hearing and balance are understandably affected.

Take sensorineural (sen-suh-ree-NOOR-ul) hearing loss, for example. It involves damage to the inner ear — the cochlea, the auditory nerve or both. Presbycusis (pres-bih-KU-sis) is the type of hearing loss that happens with aging. The hair cells in the inner ear wear out, causing the loss of sensitivity to sound. Some adults lose very little hearing as they age; others lose much more.

Other inner ear issues, like a tumor on the nerves that connect the inner ear to the brain, can cause dizziness and make balance a challenge.

This chapter outlines conditions that are linked to problems in the inner ear.

HEARING-RELATED INNER EAR ISSUES

Many inner ear conditions cause hearing loss. Here are the most common types of inner ear-related hearing loss.

Presbycusis

Presbycusis, as you just learned, is known as age-related hearing loss. Almost 1 in 10 adults ages 55 to 64 have some hearing loss. This number rises to about 1 in 3 in adults between the ages of 65 and 74. Nearly 50% of adults older than age 75 have hearing loss.

While not all people age the same way, sensory details may be a little harder to distinguish as you age. You may lose hair cells in the cochlea of the inner ear. Losing these hair cells can lead to sensorineural hearing loss. Also, your brain may lose its ability to translate signals from the auditory nerve into recognizable sounds as quickly as it used to.

At first, you may notice that you can't hear sounds that have a high frequency (pitch) as well as you used to. That's because the initial damage to hair cells often occurs where high-frequency sounds are processed. When this happens, you may not be able to hear or tell the difference between certain sounds of speech, like *ss*, *ff* and *th*.

While this is happening, the ability to hear sounds with a low frequency usually remains intact. Some sounds, like a booming bass instrument or a passing truck, may even seem *too* loud.

With presbycusis, you may also experience ringing or buzzing in your ears. This is known as tinnitus (see Chapter 5). Presbycusis also makes it hard to hold a conversation in public spaces, like in a busy store or restaurant where there's commotion and background noise.

Not being able to hear everything spoken in a conversation is much like reading a book that's had pages removed or trying to recognize a song based on just the throbbing bass line from a radio playing at your neighbor's house. It can be a frustrating, if not annoying, experience.

Presbycusis tends to run in families, which suggests that genetics is involved. Its onset may be earlier in some families than in others.

Just as it's possible to adjust to other changes that accompany aging, like vision loss, there are ways you can work with presbycusis. In particular, hearing aids can help you hear high-frequency sounds without making low-frequency sounds too loud. Hearing aids can't completely restore your hearing to what it was when you were younger, but they are helpful.

Noise-induced hearing loss

Every day, people are surrounded by noise. The bustle of traffic, the hums and grinds of machinery, people talking, music and chatter from the radio, and airplanes flying overhead are all examples. Most people probably think nothing of these familiar sounds. They generally aren't loud enough loud enough to interfere with daily routines or cause ear damage. But sometimes a noise is too loud, and some sounds may cause permanent damage.

Noise exposure can damage hearing in two ways:
- **Single explosion of noise.** Sudden, unprotected exposure to a sound measuring between 120 and 190 decibels (dB), like a rifle gunshot or

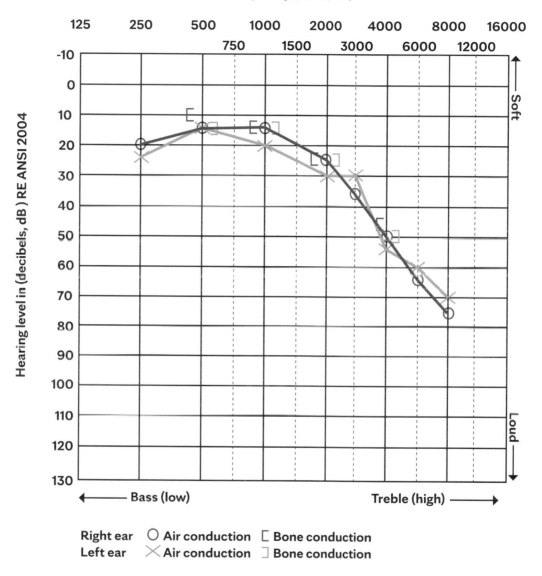

Frequency (hertz, Hz)

Hearing level in (decibels, dB) RE ANSI 2004

Bass (low)　　　Treble (high)

Right ear　　◯ Air conduction　⊏ Bone conduction
Left ear　　✕ Air conduction　⊐ Bone conduction

This audiogram shows a typical pattern of hearing loss due to presbycusis. Often with age, people typically can hear low-frequency sounds. However, it's usually harder to hear high-frequency sounds. And some high-frequency sounds may become impossible to hear, such as doorbells or bird songs.

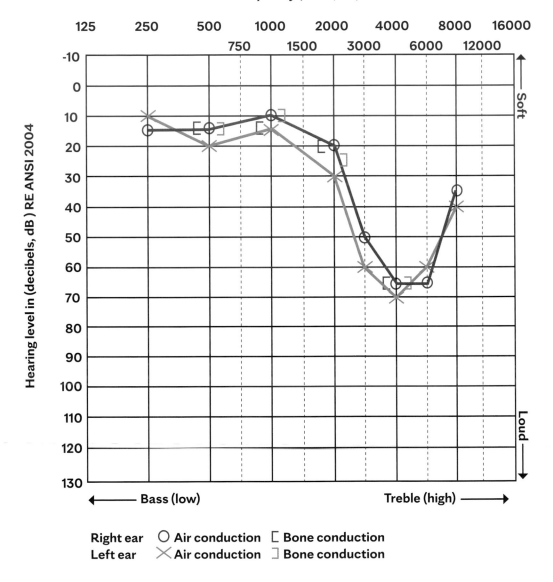

Frequency (hertz, Hz)

Hearing level in (decibels, dB) RE ANSI 2004

Soft

Loud

◄──── Bass (low)

Treble (high) ────►

| Right ear | ○ Air conduction | ⌐ Bone conduction |
| Left ear | ✕ Air conduction | ⌐ Bone conduction |

This audiogram shows a typical pattern of hearing loss due to noise. Many people are able to hear sounds at low frequencies, but their ability to hear sounds at high frequencies takes a dip, usually greatest at 4,000 hertz.

firecracker blast, can cause immediate hearing loss. The sounds of artillery and explosions are even more dangerous. Noise-induced hearing loss is a common injury in the military.

- **Prolonged exposure to loud noise.** Long-term exposure to noise levels above 85 dB can damage your hearing. This may happen at work or during recreational activities. Noise sources include power tools, lawn equipment, tractors, motorcycles and snowmobiles, and sound equipment like personal listening devices set to high volume.

Noise-induced hearing loss can occur in one or both ears. You may notice that familiar sounds seem muffled or distorted. You may also have a ringing or buzzing sensation in your ears (tinnitus).

After a sudden exposure to loud noise, you may experience these symptoms right away. But with prolonged exposure, hearing loss may be so gradual that you're not aware of it until it's pointed out to you or you have a hearing test. Plus, exposures to noise can add up over time. Loud sounds experienced years ago can contribute to hearing loss with age.

Hearing loss after noise exposure is called a temporary threshold shift.

Hearing typically returns after minutes or even days. A temporary shift that lasts beyond 30 days becomes known as a permanent threshold shift. This hearing loss is unlikely to improve.

Nearly 1 in 4 people in the United States ages 20 to 69 has some degree of hearing loss caused by exposure to loud sounds or noise at work or in leisure activities.

Preventing noise-induced hearing loss

Although noise-induced hearing loss usually can't be restored, you can prevent it. Here's how:
- Know which noises can cause damage.
- Avoid exposure to the loud noise.
- Take breaks from prolonged exposure to loud noise.
- Move away from the source of the noise.
- Wear hearing protectors when involved in loud activities.

Hearing protection is most helpful when you wear it for the entire time you're exposed to loud noise. Earplugs and earmuffs are both good options. Earplugs are small inserts that fit snugly inside the ear canal. Earmuffs fit over the entire outer ear. Each can reduce the noise by about 15 to 30 dB.

LEARN MORE

Is your hearing at risk? Learn how to protect your ears with these tips from Mayo Clinic audiologist Greta C. Stamper, Au.D., Ph.D.: links.mayoclinic.org/protectears

When earplugs and earmuffs are worn together, they offer an additional reduction of 5 dB — which is important when noise levels are high.

Whatever type of ear protection you use, make sure it's clean and it fits correctly. Earplugs should maintain an airtight seal in your ear. Earmuffs must contact the skin entirely around your ear. Devices that meet federal standards in the U.S. are available at drugstores, hardware stores, sporting goods stores and with most hearing health care providers.

U.S. companies that operate at noise levels averaging 85 dB or more over an eight-hour day are required to have a hearing conservation program. The program must include noise measurements, hearing protectors and annual hearing tests for employees, and education and training sessions.

OTHER INNER EAR PROBLEMS

Factors other than aging and noise exposure may damage the inner ear and auditory nerve, leading to problems with hearing and balance. The effects of this damage may be sudden or take shape gradually. Find common examples of inner ear-related hearing and balance problems starting on page 53 and additional balance examples in Chapter 16.

HOLD DOWN THE NOISE

Most people are aware of the dangers of work-related noise. But it's easy to overlook noise at home.

Hold down the noise level at your house with this advice:
- Turn down the volume on your television or home sound system.
- Wear snug-fitting headphones that block background noise on personal listening devices so that you don't have to turn up the volume so much.
- Choose quieter appliances.
- Place pads under noisy appliances.
- Don't run multiple appliances at the same time.
- Install carpeting to absorb sound.
- Seal windows and doors to block the noise of traffic.
- Wear earplugs or earmuffs when using power equipment.
- Rest your ears. Alternate noisy activities with quiet ones.

Hearing loss caused by recreational activities is becoming more common. Wear ear protectors when you're riding a snowmobile or motorcycle, using firearms, or listening to extremely loud music.

HOW LOUD ARE COMMON SOUNDS?

These sound levels are color-coded for easy reference to show the noises that are safe for ears (green), which sounds require caution (yellow), and which sounds can damage hearing when ear protection isn't worn (red).

Sound level (decibels)		Noise
30		Whisper
40		Refrigerator hum
50		Rainfall
60		Typical conversation, sewing machine
70		Washing machine
85		Heavy city traffic
95		Motorcycle, power lawn mower, MRI
100		Snowmobile, hand drill, blow dryer, subway train
105		Personal listening device at maximum volume
110		Chain saw, rock concert
120		Ambulance siren
130		Jet engine at takeoff
150		Firecracker
165		12-gauge shotgun
180		Rocket launch

Noises that aren't as harmful to your ears tend to fall below 60 decibels. From there, the higher the sound level, the more damage your ears can experience. Check to see which sounds you're exposed to on a regular basis and think of ways you can improve your hearing protection.

How loud is too loud? Here's a good rule of thumb: If you have to shout in order to be heard by someone an arm's length away, you're being exposed to too much noise.

Personal listening devices are more popular than ever. Their sound quality has improved over the years, and they're smaller and more convenient to use. In turn, people are spending more time listening to music and other media with these devices. Unfortunately, many users listen for too long at too high a volume. This can cause noise-induced hearing loss, which you may not notice until your ears have been significantly damaged.

Tips for using these devices: Keep the volume at a level where you can still comfortably carry on a conversation. Or use snugly fit or noise-isolating earphones. They both can help block background noise, allowing you to listen at lower decibel levels.

While you can't easily measure the decibel level of your music, a simple guideline for safe use is the 80/90 rule. This guideline says that it's OK to use a music player at 80% of maximum volume for up to 90 minutes a day. If you choose to listen for longer, the volume should be reduced. This guideline assumes that there are no additional high-level noise exposures within that 24-hour period. Many devices have a setting that allows you to prevent the volume from ever going above 80%, even when you set the volume to maximum.

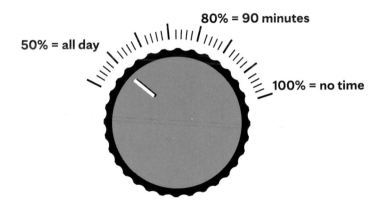

Some other ways to tell if the volume is set too high:
• You can't hear conversations going on around you.
• You find yourself shouting when you talk to people nearby.
• After listening, you experience muffled sounds or ringing in your ears.

Sudden deafness

Hearing that's lost all at once or within only a few days is known as sudden sensorineural hearing loss (SSNHL).

Between 1 and 6 out of 5,000 people experience SSNHL every year in the United States. It almost always affects just one ear. Many people notice a popping sound when it happens to them. Or they may detect the hearing loss when they first wake up or try to use the affected ear. Dizziness or tinnitus also may develop.

If you notice these symptoms, contact your doctor right away. SSNHL is often misdiagnosed as a routine ear infection or other problem. But, it can be accurately diagnosed with a good exam.

During the exam, a doctor will assess the extent of hearing loss. The less hearing loss that has occurred, the more likely it is that hearing will return within a few weeks. Although many people regain their former hearing, some may regain only some hearing in the affected ear or not regain any hearing at all.

Pinpointing the cause of SSNHL can be difficult. Most of the time, the cause is unknown. If the cause is known, taking care of the underlying problem may resolve the hearing loss.

When the cause isn't obvious, your doctor may consider many possibilities, such as:
• Viral inner ear infection
• Abrupt disruption of blood flow to the cochlea

• Membrane tear within the cochlea
• Acoustic neuroma

A special hearing test or an MRI may be done to make sure a tumor or growth isn't causing the hearing loss.

If your hearing returns quickly, you may not need treatment. If you do need treatment, your doctor may prescribe a corticosteroid like prednisone or dexamethasone to reduce the inflammation as soon as possible. Sometimes, the corticosteroid is injected directly into the middle ear through the eardrum.

It's critical to get treatment quickly. Treatment isn't as effective if it's given more than two weeks after the hearing loss. Treatment may not help at all more than six weeks later.

Viral infections

Before the widespread practice of childhood vaccinations, viruses that caused many illnesses were also responsible for hearing loss. For example, the measles virus usually attacks the cells that line the lungs and the back of the throat. Likewise, the mumps virus typically affects one of the salivary glands between the ear and the jaw. Either infection can spread to the inner ear and destroy hair cells in the cochlea, leading to hearing loss.

Hearing loss from these once-common illnesses is now rare in the United States because they can be prevented with a vaccine. Children routinely get the measles-mumps-rubella (MMR) vaccine at ages 12 to 15 months and again at 4 to 6 years. Another way to gain immunity is through natural infection with measles or mumps.

If you're traveling to a place where any of these illnesses are still prevalent, talk to your doctor to make sure your vaccinations are up to date.

Other viruses may travel by bloodstream to the cochlea, leading to hearing loss. They include the flu, chickenpox and mononucleosis viruses and cytomegalovirus (CMV).

Head trauma

A blow to the head can sometimes cause problems with hearing, especially if the part of the skull that houses the ear (temporal bone) is fractured. Such a fracture may damage the delicate structure of the cochlea or the auditory nerve. Damage to the nerve interferes with communication to the brain.

The brain rests inside the skull, protected by a cushion of spinal fluid. A sharp blow to the head will cause the brain to abruptly shift. This can tear blood vessels, pull nerve fibers and bruise tissue. Pressure waves from the blow can disrupt structures in the cochlea (damage known as a cochlear concussion) and cause sensorineural hearing loss. Hearing loss from this type of trauma may go unnoticed for some time. If you've experienced a cochlear concussion, your hearing may improve over a six-month period.

Hidden hearing loss

Some people have typical audiogram results, yet have trouble hearing in certain situations. Others have more trouble understanding than expected for a certain type of hearing loss. This is known as hidden hearing loss. People with hidden hearing loss usually have trouble understanding speech in environments with a lot of background noise but can hear sounds — even someone whispering — in a quiet room.

Historically, experts have focused on damage to hair cells or nerves in the ear as a potential cause of hidden hearing loss. The thinking is that this hearing loss is caused by the aging process and exposure to loud noises. But other, bigger issues may be at play: Loud noises can cause a loss of connections between inner hair cells and the auditory nerve (synapses). Audiograms are performed in quiet rooms, and only a few synapses are needed to hear in this situation. But if there is a lot of competing noise, the ear must try to process the sound by activating certain synapses. When these synapses are lost, signals may become more muddled, leaving the brain to struggle to understand the message.

Hidden hearing loss can also arise when certain conditions disrupt the process of cells making insulation for nerve fibers in the ear. Guillain-Barré syndrome is an example. Cognitive issues, neuropathy, head or brain injuries, stroke, attention deficit and hyperactivity disorder (ADHD), and medications also may contribute to hidden hearing loss.

Comprehensive hearing exams that go beyond an audiogram may offer a more accurate picture of what's going on. If it's possible that you have hidden hearing loss, your hearing may be tested in noisy environments. This is known as speech-in-noise testing.

Hidden hearing loss can't be treated, but reducing your exposure to loud noises, getting auditory-cognitive training, and wearing hearing aids or using other assistive devices can help manage it.

Ménière's disease

Ménière's (meh-NAYRZ) disease is characterized by spontaneous episodes of fluctuating hearing loss, tinnitus and the feeling of a plugged ear. It's often followed by a sensation of spinning or rotating (vertigo), nausea, and vomiting. One attack may last from 20 minutes to several hours, but not usually more than 24 hours. Ménière's disease can affect adults at any age, but it's most likely to occur in people in their 40s, 50s or 60s.

WHEN HEARING LOSS IS GENETIC

More than 100 genes have mutations known to cause hearing loss. About 30 of these mutations are associated with adult-onset hearing loss or progressive hearing loss. These genetic changes tend to be dominant, meaning you only have to inherit a changed gene from one parent — as opposed to inheriting a changed gene from both parents — for it to negatively affect you. Most commonly, the mutations occur in genes that are necessary for the cochlea and its sensory hair cells to work properly.

For some adults, hearing loss may be just one of many symptoms resulting from an inherited syndrome. For example, Usher's syndrome type 3 causes late-onset hearing loss, blindness and balance problems.

While genetics is known to be a fairly common cause of hearing loss in infants, much less is known about the number of adults who have inherited hearing loss. Figuring out what may be caused by genetics, what may be caused by environmental factors and what may be caused by both is difficult. Likely, there are multiple factors that contribute. However, some estimates attribute up to 55% of some forms of adult-onset hearing loss to genetic mutations. Genetics is also likely to play a part in susceptibility to age- and noise-related hearing loss, an area of research that is ongoing.

Getting a better understanding of the genetics behind hearing loss is crucial, as it could help researchers develop new therapies to prevent and treat it.

Attacks are unpredictable and can occur as often as several times a week or as infrequently as once a year. Many people say that dizziness is the worst symptom. Between attacks, many people have no symptoms at all. Although hearing comes and goes with the attacks, it may get worse over time. Ménière's disease usually affects only one ear, but some people develop symptoms in both ears.

No one knows what causes Ménière's disease, but scientists link the signs and symptoms to changes in the amount of fluid in the inner ear. Too much fluid increases pressure on the membranes of the inner ear, which may distort and occasionally rupture them. This, in turn, affects hearing and sense of balance.

Treating Ménière's disease usually involves taking medications to manage dizziness and nausea. You may also need to limit alcohol and caffeine, including chocolate, and follow a low-salt diet.

Your doctor may prescribe medication to reduce the amount of fluid in your inner ear. Examples include a water pill (diuretic), an antihistamine and a migraine medication. You may also have medications injected into the middle ear to reduce or eliminate attacks. Corticosteroids are one type of medication that may be used, because they reduce inflammation. The antibiotic gentamicin is another option. It reduces activity in the inner ear.

If dizziness is severe, inner ear surgery may be an option. Learn more about this kind of surgery on page 230.

One last note: Ménière's disease is often misdiagnosed. If you have dizziness attacks but no other symptoms, you may have another disorder, like vestibular migraine (see Chapter 14).

Labyrinthitis and vestibular neuritis

Though vestibular neuritis and labyrinthitis are similar, they're two distinct conditions. Labyrinthitis is an infection of the inner ear. Vestibular neuritis is an infection of the vestibular nerve that connects the inner ear to the brain. Both conditions may be caused by a viral infection. Lack of blood to the inner ear is another possible cause. Labyrinthitis may cause hearing loss, but vestibular neuritis does not. Here's more on both conditions.

Labyrinthitis (lab-uh-rin-THIE-tis) is an inflammation of a part of the inner ear known as the labyrinth. It can affect both the cochlea, which is vital to hearing, and the vestibular labyrinth, which plays a role in balance and eye movement. If the inflammation affects only the vestibular labyrinth, it's known as vestibular neuritis or vestibular neuronitis.

The inflammation often follows a viral infection or, more rarely, a bacterial infection. Bacterial meningitis, for example, can cause severe to profound hearing loss. Vaccinations against the organisms responsible for this infection are now routinely recommended for children and many adults.

Labyrinthitis may also occur after a blow to the head, often called a labyrinthine concussion. Or it may occur with no associated illness or trauma.

Signs and symptoms of labyrinthitis include dizziness, hearing loss, tinnitus, nausea, vomiting and involuntary movements of the eyes. Severe vertigo may last for several days. Some people lose all hearing in the affected ear.

To minimize dizziness, it's helpful to sit still and avoid sudden changes of position. Medications are sometimes used to relieve severe dizziness and nausea. Most of the time, the inflammation goes away on its own after a few weeks. Dizziness symptoms typically last no more than three days. After that period of time, it's important to resume activity so that you can adjust to any changes in function.

Treatment with antibiotics can help when the underlying problem is bacterial. Medications can relieve dizziness and nausea. If dizziness persists, some people benefit from physical or occupational therapy. Many people recover completely from labyrinthitis, but some have ongoing problems with balance and hearing loss.

The symptoms of vestibular neuritis are similar to labyrinthitis. Both cause a sudden onset of vertigo, nausea, vomiting, and involuntary, rapid and repetitive movement of the eyes (nystagmus).

Signs and symptoms of vestibular neuritis may last from several days to weeks, being severe at first and then gradually improving. Often, vestibular neuritis will develop after a cold or other upper respiratory viral infection. Most people recover completely from the neuritis, although some may experience mild imbalance after the infection has been resolved.

Prescription medications can suppress the vertigo and nausea. Steroids like prednisone help reduce inflammation from the infection. Vestibular rehabilitation is another option for recovery (see Chapter 16).

Vestibular schwannoma

A vestibular schwannoma is commonly called an acoustic neuroma. It is a benign, slow-growing tumor on the main nerve that leads from the inner ear to the brain. The tumor is the result of an uncontrolled growth of Schwann cells, which cover the nerves. An acoustic neuroma applies severe pressure on these nerves and affects their blood supply. This pressure causes hearing loss in one ear, ringing in the ear (tinnitus) and unsteadiness.

Because an acoustic neuroma affects nerves related to both hearing and balance, hearing loss and tinnitus in one ear are common in this disorder. As the tumor grows, it can affect other nerves, causing facial numbness and weakness.

Although an acoustic neuroma generally grows slowly, it can get big enough that it pushes against the brain and interferes with life-sustaining functions. Some tumors stop growing or grow so slowly that they don't need treatment. Others are removed with surgery or treated with a specialized, single dose of radiation.

To remove an acoustic neuroma, a surgeon makes a small incision behind or above the ear and removes part of the skull to reach the tumor. Once the tumor is located and removed, the bony segment is replaced to cover the opening in the skull and protect the brain.

If the tumor is removed without injuring the nerves, it's possible to maintain hearing. In general, the larger the tumor, the more likely it is that hearing, balance and facial nerves will be affected.

An acoustic neuroma can also be treated with a noninvasive treatment known as stereotactic radiosurgery. With this procedure, imaging shows where the tumor is — the location that the beams should target. The beams affect tissues only at the spot where the beams criss-cross. The beams are too weak to harm the tissue they pass through.

One of the benefits of this procedure is that the skull isn't opened. This eliminates the chances for surgical complications. And recovery time is shorter. One drawback is that this procedure isn't 100% effective. In some cases, the tumor keeps growing and needs to be removed with surgery. Even when the procedure is successful, it's typical to need MRIs to see if the tumor starts to grow again.

Reaction to medications

Certain medications or chemicals can cause hearing loss, tinnitus and balance

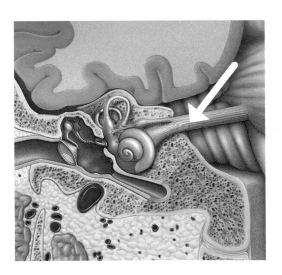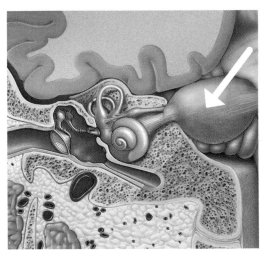

An acoustic neuroma is a tumor on the balance and hearing nerves. The arrow in the left image shows what a nerve leading from the inner ear usually looks like. The arrow in the right image shows a large tumor that has developed at the base of the bony internal auditory canal.

problems. Medications can also make existing hearing problems worse. These medications are described as ototoxic.

The effects of ototoxic medications can range from mild to severe. Effects generally depend on how much you take and how long you take the drugs. Find common ototoxic medications on page 60.

Hearing problems caused by some ototoxic drugs go away after the medication is stopped. Drugs that are known to cause permanent hearing loss are usually given only when no other option exists for treating a life-threatening disease.

More than 200 medications are considered ototoxic. If you and your doctor decide that it's in your best interest to take an ototoxic drug, an audiologist will likely test your hearing before, while and after you take the drug.

Your doctor is likely to closely monitor your hearing test results to determine how long you can continue to take the drug or when to alter the dosage.

Signs and symptoms of an ototoxic reaction include:
- Onset of tinnitus
- Worsening of existing tinnitus
- Feeling that one or both ears are plugged
- Loss of hearing or worsening of existing hearing loss
- Dizziness, sometimes with nausea and vomiting
- Loss of balance

Tell your doctor if you have an existing hearing or balance problem or if you experience inner ear problems from certain medications. This may help your doctor find ways for you to avoid unnecessary exposure to these drugs.

If you've stopped taking a medication that's caused balance issues but balance issues persist, talk to your doctor about vestibular rehabilitation. This therapy can help you adjust to and cope with an ongoing loss of balance. Learn more in Chapter 16.

Autoimmune disease

Autoimmune inner ear disease (AIED) occurs when the body's immune system mistakes ordinary cells in the inner ear for a virus or bacteria and starts attacking them. This produces an inflammatory reaction that can lead to problems with both hearing and balance. AIED is rare,

LEARN MORE

Matthew L. Carlson, M.D., Otorhinolaryngology, Mayo Clinic, explains vestibular schwannomas, a benign, slow-growing, tumor on the main nerve that leads from your inner ear to your brain, in this interview: links.mayoclinic.org/tumor

MEDICATIONS AND CHEMICALS

Listed below are some of the drugs and environmental chemicals that are known to be ototoxic. That means they can cause hearing loss. If you're taking one of these medications, it's important to keep taking it as prescribed until you talk to your doctor.

Category	Example
Salicylates	Aspirin, aspirin-containing products
Antimalarials	Chloroquine
	Quinidine sulfate
	Quinine (Qualaquin)
Antivirals and antibiotics	Azithromycin (Zithromax, others)
	Remdesivir
Loop diuretics	Bumetanide (Bumex)
	Ethacrynic acid (Edecrin)
	Furosemide (Lasix)
	Torsemide
Aminoglycoside antibiotics	Amikacin, gentamicin, neomycin, streptomycin, tobramycin
Anti-cancer drugs (anti-neoplastics)	Carboplatin, cisplatin
Environmental chemicals	Lead, manganese, n-butyl alcohol, toluene

Note that the use of alcohol can cause vertigo and nystagmus, but these symptoms are temporary and will disappear once the alcohol's effects have subsided. However, the effects of alcohol can last up to 24 hours. Prolonged alcohol misuse can damage parts of the brain and result in permanent issues with imbalance.

Effects

	Ototoxicity occurs only at high doses. Hearing loss is almost always reversible.
	Ototoxicity usually occurs only at high doses, but it can occur at lower doses. Hearing may improve when you stop using the drug.
	Ototoxicity usually occurs only at high doses, but it can occur at lower doses. Hearing usually improves when you stop using the drug.
	Ototoxicity is temporary. If these drugs are given with an ototoxic antibiotic, you may have a higher risk of permanent hearing damage.
	Risk of ototoxicity usually increases when the antibiotic is administered directly into the bloodstream. This allows the greatest amount of the drug to enter the body. Damage may be permanent.
	Drugs designed to kill cancer cells may also kill inner ear cells. The damage is often permanent and may make you more vulnerable to noise-induced hearing loss.
	Excessive exposure to these chemicals in the workplace may result in permanent hearing loss.

probably accounting for less than 1% of all cases of hearing loss. Why this reaction happens is unknown. As with many other disorders, scientists suspect that AIED may have something to do with genetics.

Hearing loss that progresses rapidly in both ears, occurring over weeks or months, is one characteristic of AIED. Sometimes, the hearing loss starts in one ear and moves to the other.

Other signs and symptoms include tinnitus, a plugged ear and, about half the time, dizziness. Because these signs and symptoms are similar to those of many other ear disorders, diagnosis can be difficult.

In addition, AIED is often associated with other autoimmune disorders, including:
• Ankylosing spondylitis, a disease that affects the spine
• Sjögren's syndrome, a condition that causes dry eyes and a dry mouth
• Cogan's syndrome, which affects the eyes and ears
• Ulcerative colitis, which affects the intestinal tract
• Wegener's granulomatosis, which inflames blood vessels
• Rheumatoid arthritis, which inflames the joints
• Scleroderma, which affects the skin and other connective tissues
• Systemic lupus erythematosus (SLE) and Behçet's syndrome, both of which can affect multiple systems in the body

If you have AIED, your doctor may prescribe oral corticosteroids (prednisone, dexamethasone) to reduce the irritation and swelling. Although corticosteroids are the most effective treatment for AIED, they have side effects that can limit long-term use. Sometimes, to prevent side effects, steroids are injected directly into the ear. Steroid therapy, especially in high doses and used for longer than three months, generally isn't recommended.

RESEARCH ON THE HORIZON

Scientists are learning more about how various aspects of health are tied to inner ear issues and how these issues may be treated and even prevented. Here's more on the latest research.

Hearing loss and cognitive decline

A growing number of studies link hearing loss to an increased risk of developing dementia, a condition that's predicted to affect up to 130 million people in the United States by 2050.

A recent review and analysis found that age-related hearing loss was significantly associated with a decline in all the main areas of cognition, including overall cognition, executive function, long-term memory and processing speed, but not an increase for certain types of dementia, such as Alzheimer's. These changes in hearing occurred up to 10 years before the onset of dementia. Separate research found that adults with hearing loss demonstrated up to a 41% more rapid rate of cognitive decline than did those without hearing loss.

Many factors can affect cognition in older adults. Some factors may be occurring at the same time, which makes determining a single cause or link tricky. For example, vascular changes may lead to both hearing loss and cognitive decline.

Plus, there may be even more to the story of hearing loss and cognitive decline — namely, what experts call the cognitive load theory. According to this theory, cognitive decline and hearing loss may be connected because the brain has to use more resources to process sounds, which leaves less energy for other cognitive tasks.

Most likely, any connection between hearing loss and dementia is influenced by many factors.

Hearing aids and cochlear implants can help those with hearing loss hear better. And some people wearing a hearing device report improvements in cognition. This may be happening because the ability to hear and understand what is being asked is improved.

Or maybe, following the cognitive load theory, being able to hear better lessens the demands on the brain and allows for more efficient processing.

Researchers continue to study the issue in hopes of finding an answer and, in turn, improved treatment options.

With all of this in mind, if you experience hearing loss, you're not guaranteed to develop dementia. At the same time, if you don't get a hearing aid or other device for your hearing loss, that doesn't mean that you'll develop cognitive issues.

Sleep apnea and hearing loss

Obstructive sleep apnea (OSA) is linked to a range of health problems — particularly those that affect the heart and circulatory system. High blood pressure, irregular heartbeats (atrial fibrillation), narrowing of blood vessels (coronary artery disease), heart failure, and heart attack, as well as diabetes and stroke, are all examples. What affects the heart is likely to affect other body functions, including hearing.

OSA happens when the throat muscles intermittently relax and block the airway during sleep. As a result, breathing stops. To make up for this, a person with OSA snores, gasps and unknowingly wakes up multiple times during the night. This, in turn, leads to daytime sleepiness. These frequent pauses in breathing reduce

LEARN MORE

Peter A. Weisskopf, M.D., and Nicholas L. Deep, M.D., Otolaryngology (ENT)/ Head and Neck Surgery, Mayo Clinic, discuss the connection between hearing and cognitive function: links.mayoclinic.org/mind oxygen levels in the blood, potentially damaging blood vessels and the heart, leading to less effective blood circulation.

The severity of OSA also appears to play a key role in the degree of hearing loss. In one study, mild OSA had no effect on hearing, while moderate OSA seemed to impact high-frequency hearing. Severe OSA had significant effects on all hearing functions in the same study.

Whether treatment for OSA through interventions such as continuous positive airway pressure (CPAP) can reduce the risk of hearing loss is unknown and warrants further investigation. However, what is known is that practicing overall healthier habits, such as eating healthy, exercising, maintaining a healthy weight and not smoking, can reduce the risk of OSA and related health problems.

Advances in treatment and prevention

For many years, researchers have been working to find therapies and a cure for hearing loss caused by damage to the inner ear (sensorineural hearing loss). While hearing aids and cochlear implants can help improve hearing, this type of hearing loss can't be reversed, and these treatments can't restore hearing to what it used to be.

Sensorineural hearing loss can't be reversed mostly because humans, unlike other animals, can't regenerate hair cells in the ears that transport sound waves to the brain, where they're processed and understood. Once hair cells are damaged

and lost, they're gone forever. And without these hair cells, you can't hear.

Scientists are learning more every day about how people hear in an effort to come up with ways to treat and reverse hearing loss. Mice are studied in this research because their ears — and the pathways between their ears and brain — are similar to those of humans.

While there's no cure yet for hearing loss, researchers are making strides in several areas. Here's what the latest studies show.

Hair cell regeneration

You learned earlier that many drugs and chemicals can cause hair cell death and, in turn, hearing loss. Loud noise, viral infections, aging and certain disorders also can cause a person to lose hair cells. Hearing loss is often linked to a loss of hair cells in the inner ear.

While it's not yet possible to regenerate hair cells after they're gone, researchers are inching closer to therapies that may one day make this possible.

Gene therapy. Gene therapy is one possible option. About 140 genes have been shown to cause deafness in humans, and more will likely be discovered. Currently, more than 3,000 clinical trials involving gene therapy are underway. Genetic issues are a major contributor in sensorineural hearing loss.

With so much known about human genes, scientists are studying how gene therapy may be used to replace lost hair cells with new, functioning hair cells. Or how gene therapy may be used to get functioning hair cells to generate new hair cells.

Gene therapy may be used to restore hearing and treat balance disorders caused by a loss of hair cells. While gene therapy shows promise in preliminary animal studies, more research is needed before it can be used in humans.

Stem cell therapy. Stem cells are the body's raw materials. They're the cells from which all other cells with specialized functions are made. Under the right conditions in the body or a lab, stem cells divide to form more cells. These cells either become new stem cells or become specialized cells with a more specific function.

One way doctors and scientists hope stem cells can be helpful is by generating healthy cells to replace diseased cells — like hair cells that are damaged and die, leading to hearing loss and balance problems. The hope is that stem cell therapy might restore hearing.

Several animal studies show that stem cells can be used to regenerate and replace hair cells in the ear. However, this therapy poses many potential risks to humans. In addition, stem cell therapy is limited due to its high cost. These challenges need to be studied and overcome before this therapy can be used in people. Still, researchers feel that this is a promising therapy. Some researchers even think that stem cell therapy and gene therapy may be used together.

Preventing damage

Researchers also are studying if medications can prevent hair cell damage in the ears. Antioxidants show promise by reducing hearing loss from loud noise. Other medications, such as citicoline, have been used to protect hearing before ototoxic drugs are used. Developing these preventives could lead to a simple pill that would reduce the risk of damage to the ears.

SOLVING INNER EAR ISSUES

For the next several decades, hearing aids and implants will remain a key focus of inner ear research. Experts will continue to refine these devices in an effort to improve quality of life for people with hearing and balance issues caused by inner ear problems.

At the same time, researchers will continue to investigate how the inner ear and its connection to the brain work. What they learn may lead to discoveries that one day completely restore hearing and perhaps prevent inner ear damage entirely.

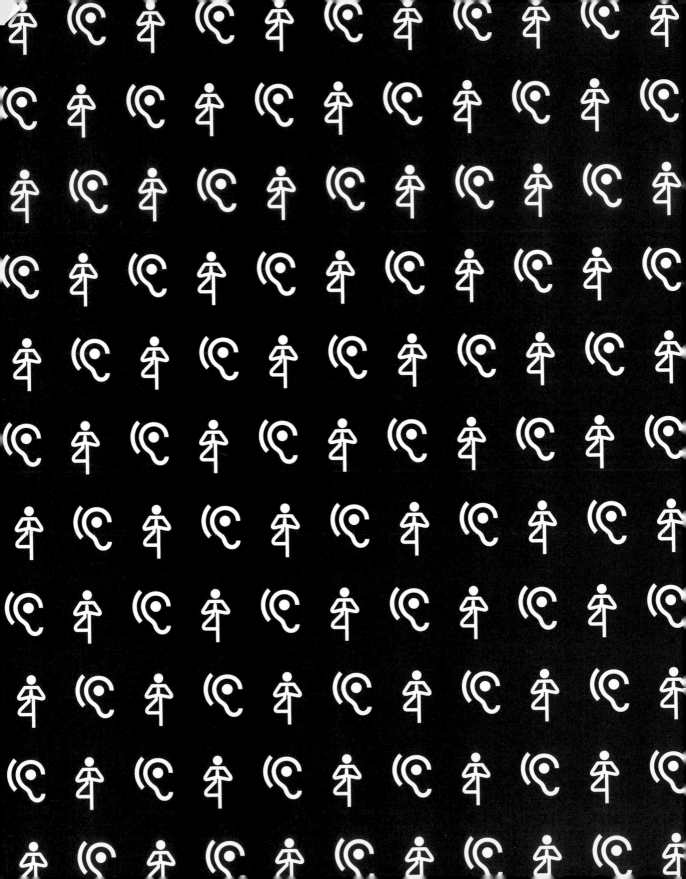

5

Tinnitus

Tinnitus (pronounced either as TIN-ih-tus or tih-NIE-tus) is the perception of sound in your ear caused by no apparent external source. The sound is characterized as a ringing, buzzing, whistling, chirping, hissing, humming, roaring or clicking, among other descriptions. Some people refer to it as music or the sound of boiling water.

Regardless of how it's described, it's a sound that's not produced in your surroundings. Often, the noise seems to originate in your head.

Many people experience brief episodes of tinnitus after being exposed to an extremely loud noise or taking certain medications. But few people are overly alarmed by such episodes, and the sound usually goes away.

According to the American Tinnitus Association, about 50 million people in the U.S. experience tinnitus. For about 20 million of these people, tinnitus is chronic, meaning it's a long-term issue. And 2% have tinnitus that's so extreme that it's almost unbearable.

The impact of tinnitus on people's lives can range anywhere from annoying to debilitating. At night, the noise may make it difficult to fall asleep. Tinnitus can also make it hard to focus on daily activities and jobs. Frustration with the unexplained sounds can often lead to anxiety, fear and depression.

Tinnitus is a symptom associated with many ear disorders as well as with other diseases, including heart disease, allergies and anemia.

UNRAVELING THE MYSTERY

What triggers tinnitus — which might explain how and why the noise occurs — is unclear. But several theories have been proposed.

One thought is that it's a phenomenon of the central nervous system, similar to the phantom-like sensations experienced after a limb amputation. A person may feel pain in his or her foot even after the leg has been removed. With tinnitus, the central auditory nervous system may be responding to the loss of hair cells in the inner ear by becoming overactive. In other words, one or more stations in the brain that process what you hear may generate abnormal activity.

In addition to too much activity in these auditory centers, parts of the brain that *aren't* involved in processing sounds also may play a role. For some people with tinnitus, for example, there seems to be a link between the auditory system and the limbic system, which is responsible for emotions like fear and anxiety. The auditory system also seems to be influenced by the part of the brain involved with touch (somatosensory system) and by the movement of body parts, like jaw clenching and certain neck movements. These movements can cause changes in the loudness and pitch of tinnitus.

Researchers have learned all of this by studying positron emission tomography (PET) scans, which reveal the parts of the brain that are used to accomplish specific tasks. PET images of the brains of people with tinnitus are leading researchers to

think that parts of the brain that process what people hear interact with areas of the brain that aren't involved in hearing. This may explain why some people with tinnitus perceive the sounds they hear more intensely compared with others who have tinnitus.

Other researchers think the cause of tinnitus may lie with the activity of chemicals in the auditory nerve. These chemicals carry messages from the inner ear to the brain. Finally, for some people, tinnitus may stem from turbulent blood flow through arteries and veins that lie close to the inner ear.

While there are many possible explanations, scientists agree that tinnitus is a complex systemwide problem that involves the parts of the central nervous system that process sounds — and many parts that don't.

The good news is that tinnitus generally isn't serious or life-threatening. In a few cases, tinnitus may even be caused by an underlying condition that's treatable.

While there's usually no cure for tinnitus, there are many ways to manage it and lessen its effect on your daily life. You may need your doctor and an audiologist, and your participation is critical. Later in this chapter, you'll learn several ways to manage symptoms of tinnitus.

TYPES OF TINNITUS

Descriptions of tinnitus vary greatly from one person to the next. The only thing they have in common seems to be the existence of an unexplained noise in the head or ears.

Some experts have categorized the condition into two broadly defined types: objective and subjective.

Objective tinnitus

Objective tinnitus, sometimes called pulsatile (PUL-suh-tile) tinnitus, is a sound that can be heard by other people as well as by you. The sounds originate within your body, most commonly from turbulent blood flow in your arteries and veins. Very few people with tinnitus have this type.

If you have atherosclerosis, for example, a buildup of cholesterol and other fatty deposits causes your blood vessels to lose elasticity. This restricts the vessels from flexing slightly with each heartbeat. Narrower openings require a more forceful blood flow. Your heart works harder — to the point where your ears

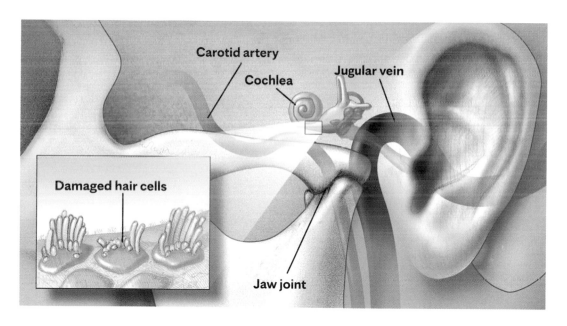

Tinnitus can develop from multiple causes. For example, some researchers think that damage to the hair cells in the cochlea leads to overactivity in the part of the nervous system that processes sounds. Blood vessels like the carotid artery and the jugular vein may be another culprit. They're close to the inner ear, so turbulent blood flow through these blood vessels may produce a sound. Tinnitus may also result from a misalignment of the jaw joint (temporomandibular joint), head or neck trauma, or a variety of other medical conditions.

can detect each heartbeat. Your doctor may hear the sound with the help of a stethoscope.

High blood pressure can make objective tinnitus more noticeable. So can factors that temporarily increase blood pressure, such as stress, alcohol or caffeine use, and high amounts of sodium in your diet. Repositioning your head usually can cause the sounds to disappear.

Poorly formed small blood vessels (capillaries) connecting your arteries and

TINNITUS AND SLEEP APNEA

The trademark ringing of tinnitus — or in some cases buzzing, roaring, clicking, hissing, or humming — can significantly affect sleep. People with tinnitus may experience insomnia and related signs and symptoms, including fatigue, irritability and problems concentrating. Some experts have suggested that tinnitus may be linked to other sleep issues, too, like sleep apnea. Sleep apnea causes people to periodically stop breathing as they sleep, reducing oxygen in the blood and causing them to awaken frequently during the night.

Not much research has been done on the connection between sleep apnea and tinnitus. A study conducted in Taiwan found that middle-aged and older people who had sleep issues — particularly sleep apnea — were more likely to have tinnitus than those without sleep problems. However, the study couldn't prove if one caused the other.

In some cases, other health conditions may be the culprit. For example, anything that increases pressure in the brain (intracranial hypertension) can cause tinnitus and sleep apnea to occur together. Sleep disturbances and tinnitus may also share common neurological causes, like an overactive nervous system.

One study found that people with bothersome tinnitus have more activity in an area of the brain that controls emotions (the amygdala). In turn, this suggests that people with bothersome tinnitus have stronger emotional responses to the sounds of tinnitus than do those whose tinnitus is not bothersome. A chronic lack of sleep caused by sleep apnea may make these responses more intense and worsen the way people view their tinnitus.

Treatments used to treat sleep apnea, including continuous positive airway pressure (CPAP) therapy, can improve quality of sleep and lessen fatigue.

veins also can produce a pulse that others can hear. Other sources of objective tinnitus include muscle spasms, movement of the eustachian tube and spontaneous vibrations of hair cells.

Treating the underlying disorder may help reduce or even eliminate the sounds. That's why it's important to describe the tinnitus to your doctor and receive an accurate diagnosis. Be as specific as you can about the noises you hear and under what circumstances they occur.

Subjective tinnitus

Subjective tinnitus is the most common type of tinnitus. It involves sounds that only you detect. Scientists aren't sure what causes these sounds. To study the problem, they must depend on how well people describe what they're hearing.

Still, experts agree that subjective tinnitus starts within the structures of the inner ear, the central auditory pathways or elsewhere in the brain.

Although the cause of subjective tinnitus remains unclear, experts think that several factors can contribute to the condition or make it worse.

Here are some of the most common causes of subjective tinnitus.

Hearing loss

Exposure to loud noise, even for a short time, can damage the hair cells in your cochlea and cause permanent hearing loss. Most people with tinnitus have some form of hearing loss. It's more common for those with noise-induced hearing loss. It may be that the damage to hair cells also causes the tinnitus.

Some researchers believe that age-related hearing loss (presbycusis) also may play a role in tinnitus. As presbycusis muffles sounds from the outside world, tinnitus may become more noticeable. Other conditions that can reduce hearing, like impacted earwax or ear infection, also may increase awareness of tinnitus.

HOW TO DESCRIBE TINNITUS

Here are several ways you may describe the noises you hear:
- Ringing
- Buzzing
- Roaring
- Clicking
- Hissing
- Humming
- Pulsing or a heartbeat

Medications

More than 650 drugs are associated with tinnitus. Some of these drugs can injure the ear (ototoxic), sometimes permanently. These prescriptions are usually given only when absolutely necessary, such as for significant illnesses like cancer.

Other drugs can produce tinnitus as a side effect. That's why it's always important to discuss potential side effects of any medication with your doctor. After you start taking a drug, tell your doctor if your hearing is reduced or if you experience tinnitus. Stopping the drug or adjusting the dosage often eliminates the problem. If you already have tinnitus, be sure to tell your doctor.

Jaw disorders

Researchers have found a strong relationship between tinnitus and temporomandibular joint disorders. A misaligned joint connecting your jaw and the temporal bone of your skull may cause clicking or grating noises whenever you move your jaw. A dentist who specializes in treating this joint may be able to correct this.

Other factors

Various conditions or lifestyle factors may cause tinnitus:
- Exposure to excessive noise
- Serious trauma or injury to the head or neck

HYPERACUSIS

Hyperacusis (hi-pur-uh-KOO-sis) is another condition that's often associated with tinnitus. Hyperacusis involves a heightened aversion to sound. It happens when everyday noise, like traffic, conversation or a telephone ring, seems uncomfortably loud. Like the cause of tinnitus, what causes hyperacusis is unknown.

Hyperacusis may be even more debilitating than tinnitus. A person with severe hyperacusis may avoid social situations for fear of painful noise exposure (phonophobia), choosing instead to stay in a secluded environment. Although some form of hyperacusis may occur in people with hearing loss, those reporting hyperacusis usually don't have problems hearing.

Treatment consists of counseling and participating in a program that gradually increases the tolerance of everyday sounds. This may involve a white noise generator — an electronic device that generates a persistent hissing sound similar to what you may hear when a radio is tuned between stations. Initially the device is tuned to a level you can barely hear and then gradually increased to higher levels over time.

QUESTIONS YOU MAY BE ASKED

Before talking with your doctor about your tinnitus, prepare yourself by answering these questions, which doctors often ask:

- Is one ear affected or both? ☐ One ear ☐ Both ears
- If only one ear is affected, which one is it? ☐ Right ear ☐ Left ear
- Do you have hearing loss? ☐ Yes ☐ No
- Do you have any other symptoms that come along with the noise, such as ear fullness, dizziness or headache?
- Does the noise come and go, or is it always there?
- What does the noise sound like? (See page 71 for examples of descriptions you may use.) _____

_____

_____

_____

- Is the noise high-pitched or low-pitched? ☐ High-pitched ☐ Low pitched
- How loud is the noise? ☐ Fairly quiet ☐ Somewhat loud ☐ Very loud
- Are the sounds constant, or do they change in loudness or pitch? ☐ Constant ☐ Changing
- What circumstances make the tinnitus better or worse?

_____

_____

_____

- How does this condition affect your work habits and your ability to sleep and to concentrate?

_____

_____

_____

_____

_____

- How has this condition affected your stress level?

_____

_____

_____

_____

_____

- Schwannomas (shwah-NO-muhs), which are benign tumors that grow on the fibers of the balance and hearing nerves
- A stiffening of the ossicle bones in the middle ear (otosclerosis)
- Ménière's disease, which causes excess fluid in the inner ear
- Too much sodium in the diet
- Stress, either emotional or physical

DIAGNOSIS

There's little doubt that tinnitus can be troublesome. In many cases, tinnitus triggers a cycle of growing discomfort: Annoyance leads to increased attention to the noise, which causes greater frustration. Some people find the distraction so severe that they're unable to carry on with their regular daily activities.

Several options are available that may allow you to manage tinnitus and still function in life with a reasonable degree of comfort.

First, talk about the condition with your physician or audiologist. He or she can help identify or rule out a treatable cause of your tinnitus. Other specialists may become involved in the diagnosis. If an underlying condition is causing the

tinnitus, treating the cause may resolve the tinnitus. Measures such as treating an ear infection or removing impacted earwax also may help reduce tinnitus.

If the cause of your tinnitus is unknown, you and your medical team can decide how best to treat your symptoms. A medical history, physical exam, hearing tests and lab tests may provide vital clues. In addition to making these assessments, an audiologist may try to determine the specific frequency (pitch) and intensity (loudness) of your tinnitus through audiological tests. This information can help you and your medical team select the best treatment for your situation.

TREATMENT OPTIONS

Though many questions remain about tinnitus, several strategies can help you manage its signs and symptoms, manage your daily responsibilities and lead a fulfilling life.

You and your medical team may try several approaches — including counseling and various treatments — before deciding which one works best for you. It's often helpful to use more than one strategy. Here are several approaches.

LEARN MORE

Get additional expert insight on tinnitus in this interview with Gayla L. Poling, Ph.D., a Mayo Clinic audiologist, in this podcast:
links.mayoclinic.org/tinnitus

Hearing aids

Since most people with tinnitus also have hearing loss, one treatment approach involves wearing hearing aids. Hearing aids may reduce your perception of tinnitus and help you hear better. Programmed for your hearing loss, hearing aids make environmental sounds louder, helping to make tinnitus less noticeable. Many people who have hearing loss and tinnitus say that their tinnitus diminishes when they wear hearing aids.

If you don't have hearing loss, hearing aids can also be used to produce a low-level background masking noise that's usually easier to tolerate than tinnitus is. Even if you don't have trouble hearing, you may benefit from the addition of subtle background noise to cover (mask) the sounds of tinnitus. These sounds usually resemble static noise or wind chimes.

With hearing aids, you may have controls to adjust the loudness of sounds, but the frequency is usually programmed by your audiologist to achieve the best effect.

Before committing to buying hearing aids, confirm that they can provide enough benefit to make them worth the investment. Ask your hearing health care provider about the return policy in case hearing aids aren't the answer for you.

Other masking sources

Tinnitus maskers are devices worn behind or in the ears. They look like hearing aids, but instead of making environmental sounds louder, they produce low-level background noise that may be easier to tolerate than the sounds of tinnitus are.

With current tinnitus maskers, you can adjust the loudness. In some cases, you can select from several types of noise to obtain the most benefit. Some systems must be programmed by an audiologist.

Often, tinnitus is most noticeable at night. Some people find it helpful to use a bedside masker to play soothing sounds, like ocean waves, falling rain and white noise, as they prepare to sleep. These sounds help with relaxation and obscure tinnitus during sleep. You can find maskers as stand-alone devices or as apps for your cellphone or tablet.

Drug therapy

Although there are no medications that can cure tinnitus, some may help lessen its effects.

Tricyclic antidepressants (amitriptyline and nortriptyline), for example, have been used to treat tinnitus with some success. These medications are generally used for only severe tinnitus, as they can cause troublesome side effects, including dry mouth, blurred vision, constipation and heart problems.

Alprazolam (Xanax) also may help reduce tinnitus symptoms. However, it can cause drowsiness and nausea and can become habit-forming.

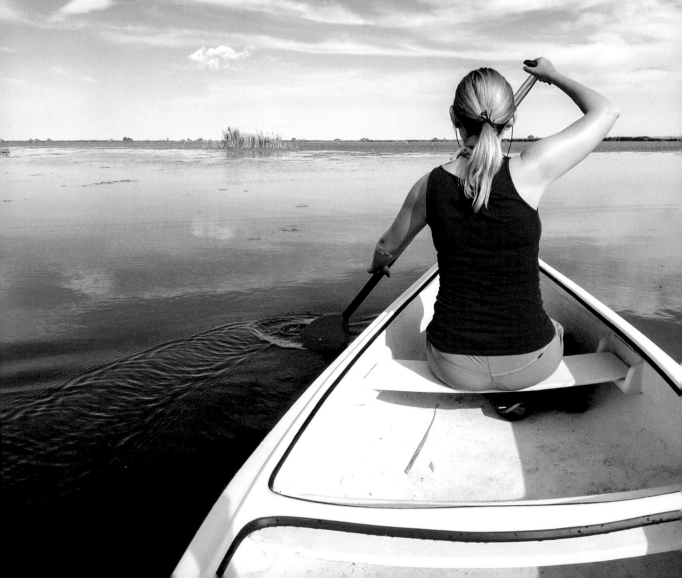

"**Distract yourself.** Many people say they don't hear tinnitus if they're not paying attention to it. Do things that you enjoy and that absorb your attention. This will help take your mind off the tinnitus and provide needed relief."

SELF-HELP TIPS FOR TINNITUS

Reduce the severity of tinnitus and cope with its symptoms by taking these steps:

Protect your hearing. Avoid loud noises, which may decrease your hearing and worsen tinnitus. If you work in a noisy environment, wear hearing protection devices regularly.

Fill your environment with sound. If you're in a quiet setting where tinnitus may seem more obvious, use a masker, fan, soft music, low-volume radio or commercially available sound generator to produce soft background noise that masks the tinnitus. Listening to pleasant and relaxing sounds can be helpful.

Distract yourself. Many people say they don't hear tinnitus if they're not paying attention to it. Do things that you enjoy and that absorb your attention. This will help take your mind off the tinnitus and provide needed relief.

Manage your stress. Stress can make tinnitus seem worse. The basic principles of a healthy lifestyle go a long way toward reducing stress — get plenty of sleep and exercise, and eat a healthy diet. For example, reducing tobacco, alcohol, caffeine and salt intake may help you better cope with the aggravation of your tinnitus.

Practice good sleep habits. People who sleep well tend to manage their tinnitus better. Although you might not be able to control all the factors that interfere with sleep, you can adopt habits that encourage better sleep. For example, try to go to bed and wake up at roughly the same time every day, and keep your bedroom comfortable and dark.

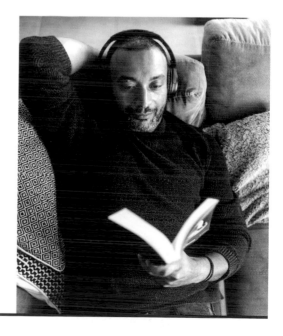

Educate yourself. Learning about tinnitus can give you a sense of control over it. Resources such as the American Tinnitus Association are listed at the back of this book.

Tinnitus retraining therapy

Tinnitus retraining therapy (TRT) is based on the idea that a person can gradually lose the awareness of a sound if that sound poses no threat or demands little attention. People can become oblivious to the sound of a ticking clock or whirring fan, even a passing train. But if the sound carries some sort of meaning with it — for example, you associate a ticking clock with being late or behind schedule — it's likely to heighten your awareness and may make the sound less stressful.

This concept is applied to coping with tinnitus. If you have tinnitus, you may have a constant urge to examine the sounds and find a cause for what you're hearing. Being unable to identify a source may leave you feeling frustrated and insecure, which further focuses your attention on the tinnitus. When this happens, it may seem as though you'll never lose your awareness of the sounds.

The goal of TRT is to get you accustomed to the tinnitus so that its steady, persistent sound becomes just like other nonthreatening sounds and blends into the background. If the effort is successful, you'll perceive tinnitus less often on a conscious level. TRT uses a combination of sound therapy and counseling.

To start treatment, you may be fit with noise generators in both ears and asked to wear them all day. The devices are set such that the generated soft noise is audible but doesn't mask your tinnitus. In other words, the generated noise and the tinnitus blend together.

You'll also receive counseling that helps you perceive the tinnitus in a way that no longer causes fear or obsession. The audiologist will explain what's known about tinnitus and how you can get used to the sound.

This therapy takes time. Most people participate in the program for one or two years before stopping the use of the noise generators. Although TRT isn't for everyone, most people undergoing this treatment report at least some success in reducing their perception of tinnitus.

Integrative therapy

Integrative therapy encompasses treatments that are used alongside other, more mainstream options. Integrative treatment has typically been offered in a "when all else fails" approach. However, ideally, any such treatment would be incorporated from the beginning into a program designed to address all aspects of tinnitus management.

Like other therapies used for tinnitus, research hasn't proved that integrative options will offer benefit. It's important to remember that there is no cure for tinnitus, and most treatments focus on coping with the effects. However, using one or more of the following may offer relief.

Acupuncture

Acupuncture involves the insertion of very thin needles into the skin at strategic points on the body in an attempt to rebalance energy flow. Performed by a licensed acupuncturist trained in traditional Chinese medicine, acupuncture is individually tailored — to the person's age, lifestyle and body type, for example — and focused on treating the whole person. For people with tinnitus, common spots to place needles include in front of the ear and behind the ear lobe.

Acupuncture has been shown to benefit some conditions, including knee arthritis, tension headaches, and nausea and vomiting linked to chemotherapy. But the research gets a little murky when it comes to whether this treatment helps reduce the impact of tinnitus. Older studies either found no benefit or had flaws in their research designs that made it difficult to determine acupuncture's true effects. Some studies did seem to find at least some benefit if people perceived it was working or expected that acupuncture would help.

Biofeedback

Biofeedback is a form of relaxation that helps people tune into body functions and learn how to control them. The ultimate goal is to help people change their reactions to tinnitus, thereby reducing stress caused by tinnitus.

A special biofeedback device gathers information from the body, such as heart rate or breathing rate, and displays it. Effectively, this shows how the body reacts to stress. This information can be used to make changes in how a person reacts to stress, which can lower stress levels. Many people with tinnitus report a reduction in their symptoms after they successfully change how they respond to them.

Cognitive behavioral therapy

Cognitive behavioral therapy helps people explore and process thoughts and emotions related to their physical tinnitus symptoms and behaviors. This is important given how many people experience distress because of tinnitus — and how distress may worsen the condition and, possibly, be a cause for tinnitus.

Sessions are typically led by a psychotherapist or other licensed mental health professional. The provider often asks about a person's history of tinnitus — how it started, the ways it affects the individual and the negative impacts it's causing, for example. The psychotherapist can then help to identify and reshape a person's beliefs about his or her condition and negative thoughts associated with it (cognitive restructuring). Sometimes, people have misconceptions about tinnitus that need clearing up, such as a belief that tinnitus is damaging their hearing or is a sign of mental illness.

Therapists can then help come up with coping mechanisms, including how to use distractions and relaxation techniques. People using cognitive behavioral therapy typically keep a diary and do homework exercises. Therapy may be done in person or online with a trained therapist. Both ways are effective.

Cognitive behavioral therapy isn't likely to reduce the perception of how loud tinnitus is or any associated depression, but research has shown that it can help manage the condition and improve quality of life. Of all the integrative therapy options, cognitive behavioral therapy is the only one that's routinely recommended, based on research.

Health coaching

Health coaching focuses on the relationship between health care providers and people with tinnitus, with the providers offering education and counseling on tinnitus and how to manage it. People learn more about tinnitus — including how it may develop and which treatments may help. The last part is especially important. Frustration with tinnitus can drive some people to try just about any treatments, including dubious ones.

Education may include brochures on tinnitus, recommendations for self-help books that focus on specific management techniques and resources that detail treatment options, like cognitive behavioral therapy and sound therapy. In some cases, referrals to another health care provider, like a psychologist or audiologist, may be needed.

Education and coaching can improve quality of life and how well people cope with tinnitus.

Mindfulness meditation

Mindfulness meditation trains you to be aware of what's going on inside your mind — feelings, thoughts, sensations, urges — while also teaching you to separate an event (hearing tinnitus sounds) from reactions to the event (feeling frustrated or upset about hearing the sound). A specific type of mindfulness meditation called mindfulness-based relaxation training uses meditation and yoga to promote awareness and reduce stress.

Research has found that mindfulness therapies are effective for treating

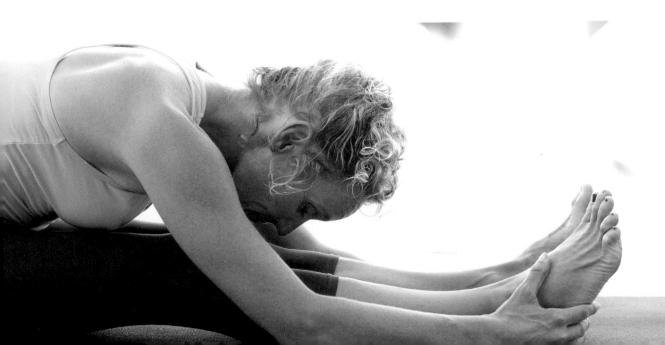

THE STRESS-TINNITUS CONNECTION

Tinnitus causes stress — that's a fact that's probably not surprising given how disruptive tinnitus can be to everyday life. Up to 60% of people with tinnitus report long-term emotional distress. But what's not as clear is which comes first, the tinnitus or the stress. Could stress be responsible for the development of tinnitus or the worsening of it?

The answer isn't entirely clear, although some experts have noted that it's common for people to report that they had psychological distress before or during the onset of tinnitus. One study compared people experiencing high levels of stress to those who were exposed to loud noises at their jobs and found that the probability of developing tinnitus was about the same between the two groups. If people were stressed and exposed to loud noises, their risk of developing tinnitus doubled.

Tinnitus is thought to be strongly influenced by how a person processes emotional stimuli, and it often appears alongside other mental health issues, like depression and anxiety. Some experts think that people who experience worsening or disabling tinnitus are those who tend to react the most strongly to unpleasant sounds. In turn, they may be unable to "shut off" or effectively cope with stressors to lessen their negative impact.

In people with distressful tinnitus, images of the brain show that these responses tend to be centered in the emotional center of the brain (amygdala), while people who have lower levels of tinnitus distress tend to bypass the amygdala and use parts of the brain responsible for problem-solving and judgment instead.

Because there's likely a psychological component to tinnitus, addressing mental health through treatment with techniques like cognitive behavioral therapy is key to managing tinnitus. As you learned earlier, cognitive behavioral therapy often involves interventions focused on changing negative thoughts and feelings about tinnitus, cutting out negative coping mechanisms, and increasing positive ways of coping.

In research focused on cognitive behavioral therapy as a treatment for tinnitus, study participants reported significant improvements in quality of life and depression following therapy. It didn't change the volume of tinnitus they were experiencing, but it helped them cope with it. Medication used to help treat symptoms of anxiety and stress also may be helpful.

conditions that, like tinnitus, cause distress. Chronic pain is one example. In small pilot studies focused on tinnitus, mindfulness meditation led to positive changes in several areas, including how severe people felt their tinnitus was.

TREATMENT OPTIONS UNDER STUDY

Currently, tinnitus treatments are focused on helping people cope with perceived sounds. To date, no treatment has been shown to reduce or eliminate the sound of tinnitus.

Research into therapies is ongoing. Some treatments have shown promise but require more research to prove they're safe and effective. Other studies haven't panned out, but the results of these studies may help fuel new, more promising research down the road. Here are several areas of research currently under study.

Neuromodulation

Most potential electrical stimulation (neuromodulation) therapies being tested to treat tinnitus are based on the theory that tinnitus is a central nervous system disorder.

When the cochlea is subjected to trauma (such as from noise), it's thought that neurons in various parts of the brain become more active and fire together to make up for damage in cochlear hair cells, which may lead to the development of tinnitus. Research has focused on whether electrical stimulation might help decrease activity or alter these pathways and thus decrease tinnitus symptoms.

Stimulation occurs via devices placed outside the head (noninvasive) or surgically implanted inside the head (invasive).

Noninvasive techniques

Two main types of noninvasive stimulation for tinnitus are under study. Here's how they work and how well they work.

Transcranial magnetic stimulation

During this procedure, an electromagnetic coil attached to a stimulation machine is placed against the scalp and painlessly delivers magnetic pulses — anywhere between 100 and 3,000 — in a rhythmic fashion. This produces a magnetic field that passes through the cranium. These pulses are thought to reduce activity in parts of the brain that may be overactive in people with tinnitus.

Some studies showed improvement in tinnitus severity. This procedure also appeared to suppress tinnitus. However, these studies had flaws, including small numbers of participants and problems with study design. Randomized controlled trials have shown no difference in improvement in tinnitus severity or quality of life when comparing those receiving the treatment to those receiving the placebo. Also, the long-term effects of magnetic stimulation aren't known. For these reasons, transcranial magnetic stimulation isn't regularly recommended to treat tinnitus.

Transcranial direct current stimulation
Transcranial direct stimulation uses electrodes attached to a battery-powered device. The electrodes are covered by wet sponges and placed over the scalp to deliver a weak but constant current to various parts of the brain to decrease neuron activity.

In studies, this treatment temporarily reduced tinnitus volume and distress anywhere from seconds to hours. How long the benefits lasted depended on the part of the brain being treated. This treatment also showed some promise for conditions that commonly occur alongside tinnitus, including anxiety and depression. No standard regimen exists yet for this form of treatment, and while it shows promise in alleviating tinnitus and associated conditions, more research is needed.

Invasive techniques

Some implanted devices are under study for their potential in treating tinnitus. Here's how each technique works — and what researchers have learned about each method's effectiveness.

Deep brain stimulation The goal of deep brain stimulation is to modify or disrupt the circuits in the brain responsible for processing tinnitus sounds.

This treatment involves surgically implanting an electrode on the opposite side of the brain from the tinnitus symptoms. For those people experiencing tinnitus in both ears, the electrode would be implanted on the right side of the head, or the nondominant side of the brain.

Deep brain stimulation is effective for people who have treatment-resistant forms of conditions like tremors, Parkinson's disease and chronic pain. However, electrodes aren't implanted solely to relieve tinnitus, so research has focused on deep brain stimulation's impact on tinnitus in people with movement disorders. Tinnitus in these people doesn't represent tinnitus in people who are otherwise healthy, so research results likely can't be applied to the typical person with tinnitus. Study participants reported lower tinnitus volume when the stimulation was turned on, but more research is needed.

Cochlear implant Designed to treat significant hearing loss, a cochlear implant bypasses the inner ear to directly stimulate the hearing nerve. In theory, this could help people with tinnitus, who are thought to experience changes in their brains' circuitry. The key components of the implant are a microphone and sound processor behind the ear to pick up sounds, a decoding chip placed under the skin to transmit information from the microphone, and electrodes connected directly to the brainstem that alert to sound when stimulated.

Research suggests that many people who received a cochlear implant experienced positive changes to their tinnitus. Usually, this meant a reduction in loudness.

Vagus nerve stimulation One vagus nerve runs down each side of the body, from the brainstem through the neck, chest and belly. It's responsible for calming the nervous system following a fight-or-flight response in stressful situations. Previous research has shown that stimulating this nerve can treat conditions such as epilepsy and depression. Researchers are looking into what impact it may have on tinnitus.

Vagus nerve stimulation delivers electrical impulses to the vagus nerve via a nerve stimulator. Traditionally, this device is surgically implanted under the skin on the chest and a wire is threaded under the skin to connect the device to the left vagus nerve. When activated, the device sends electrical signals along the left vagus nerve to the brainstem, which then sends signals to certain areas in the brain. There are also noninvasive vagus nerve stimulation devices that don't require surgical implantation.

Preliminary research has shown that pairing nerve stimulation with sound therapy may help improve auditory processing and, by default, reduce stress and disability caused by tinnitus. However, research is in the very early stages. So far, it appears that this type of nerve stimulation may not have many benefits without sound therapy.

Lidocaine

Lidocaine is best known as a form of anesthesia that blocks pain. However, it's also been studied in the treatment of tinnitus based on its ability to alter the tinnitus pathway.

Several factors make lidocaine a less-than-ideal treatment for tinnitus. First, it's typically not convenient to administer, because it requires either an injection or an IV. And any benefit is often short-lived at best and may not outweigh the risk of side effects, including vertigo, nausea and vomiting.

A recent pilot study investigated whether a lidocaine patch placed on the skin could provide greater — and more convenient — benefits with minimal side effects. While this study was promising, many participants dropped out, citing that the benefits didn't outweigh the high cost of the patches.

Neuromonics

A neuromonics program uses counseling and listening to music that's embedded with background noise to gradually desensitize people to tinnitus. The therapy is performed up to four hours a day, from 6 to 24 months. Over time, the background noise is reduced, which is thought to lead to desensitization.

The benefits of a neuromonics program aren't known because no unbiased and independent research exists to clearly show how well it works.

Marijuana (cannabis)

Cannabis is the generic term for drugs derived from the plants in the Cannabis genus. Cannabis has more than 400 chemicals, including delta-9-tetrahydrocannabinol (THC) and cannabidiol (CBD). THC is associated with "feel good" feelings produced by marijuana and contains anti-nausea, anti-inflammatory, anti-pain and antioxidant properties. CBD does not alter mood but is linked to anti-seizure, anti-anxiety and sedative properties.

Given these traits, it's been hypothesized that cannabis could reduce overactivity in the brain associated with tinnitus. Research in this area is lacking, however, and has mainly been performed on animals. In many studies, cannabis was found to trigger or worsen tinnitus.

Ketamine

Most often used for diagnostic and surgical procedures, ketamine is a controlled substance that has been studied for use in treating short-term tinnitus via injection in the ear. Animal and initial human studies showed promise. However, large-scale studies failed to show that the treatment was effective. The potential side effects of ketamine (sometimes referred to as special K when used illegally as a recreational drug) include hallucinations, confusion, agitation and potential for abuse.

Diet

Various multivitamins (such as B vitamins), zinc, antioxidants, and herbal remedies, including *Ginkgo biloba* and melatonin, have been touted as tinnitus treatments. However, research hasn't shown that any supplement is effective. Also, some of these remedies can be costly and may interact with prescription medications.

Tinnitus can be frustrating to understand and live with, but by learning about it and exploring the many options available, there are ways you can cope with the stress and frustration it can cause and lessen its effects on your life.

Hearing 101

PART 3

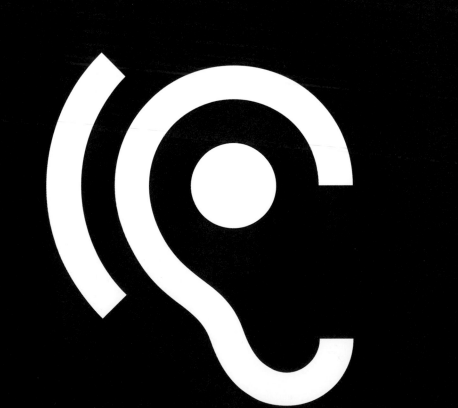

6

How you hear

Now that you've learned a little bit about the most common hearing and balance issues, let's take a deep dive into the mechanics of the ear and what can cause these issues in the first place.

In this chapter and the next, you'll get a behind-the-scenes look at how you hear and what happens during a hearing exam.

CHARACTERISTICS OF SOUND

The ear is a series of delicate, complex structures that enables you to collect and make sense of sound. But what is sound exactly?

Sound occurs whenever a substance — or, really, the molecules that make up the substance — vibrates. When a substance vibrates, it displaces all the molecules around it, much like how, when you throw a rock into a pond, it causes the water to ripple in every direction. A vibration moves from molecule to molecule in the form of a sound wave.

You hear sound waves that travel through air, like the clap of an audience's applause at the end of a performance or the hum of pistons and belts in a running car engine.

Sounds also travel through fluid. For example, you can hear the splashes of nearby swimmers when you're underwater at a pool. Sounds travel through solid matter like bone or steel, too. The thump you hear when you bump your head against an object is partly a result of vibrations traveling through your skull, as well as through air.

When a sound wave travels through the air to your outer ear and reaches your eardrum, it triggers a chain reaction through the ossicles, cochlea, auditory nerve and brain that allows you to hear the sound.

As you know, one sound can be vastly different from another. Think of the low-pitched rumble of a diesel truck and the high-pitched whine of a lightweight motorbike. Both sounds come from a combustion engine. But there's no mistaking one sound for the other. The differences between sounds arise mainly from three qualities — frequency, intensity and timbre. The first two qualities can be measured, and the third is subjective. Here's more on each.

Frequency

The frequency of sound, also known as pitch, is how often a sound wave fluctu-ates within a given period of time. It's usually measured in cycles per second, called hertz (Hz). The more fluctuations per second, the higher the frequency.

Sound frequencies that humans can hear range from around 20 Hz, a very low pitch, to 20,000 Hz, a very high pitch. Common sounds in human speech cover a broad range, from near 250 Hz (a low-pitched vowel sound such as *ooo*) to 4,000 to 6,000 Hz (a high-pitched consonant sound such as *ss* or *ff*).

Intensity

The intensity of sound is measured by its loudness (amplitude). This quality is associated with the level of disturbance of the sound wave. It's measured in decibels (dB).

For example, a hushed whisper might be measured at 30 decibels sound pressure

PITCH

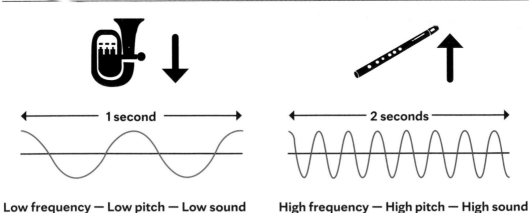

1 second	2 seconds
Low frequency — Low pitch — Low sound	High frequency — High pitch — High sound

level (dB SPL). A gunshot, on the other hand, might register at 140 to 170 dB SPL. Noise at this intensity is too loud for the human ear to tolerate, especially when you're exposed to it for a long time. Sounds that are too loud can cause permanent damage if the ears aren't protected with earplugs or a hearing protective device (earmuffs).

When you say a noise is too soft, comfortably loud or painfully loud, you're describing the sound's intensity.

Timbre

The most subjective aspect of sound might be its timbre (TAM-bur). Timbre describes the quality of sound. It allows you to tell the difference between sounds of the same frequency and intensity, like the same note played by different musical instruments or the same consonant or vowel spoken by different voices.

The tone of a piccolo or flute, for example, vibrates within a restricted range of frequencies. This tone would be represented by a relatively smooth, rolling waveform.

The timbre of a saxophone or piano is more complex. Their multiple vibrations, at many different frequencies, are represented by a jagged waveform. The dissonant ping from dropping a wooden pencil on a hard floor is another example of a complex sound.

SOUND PATHWAYS

Sound is created by molecular vibrations moving through matter. Hearing is the perception of that sound. When you hear a sound, you perceive its frequency, intensity and timbre all at once.

While the journey of a sound wave through the ear and to your brain

AMPLITUDE

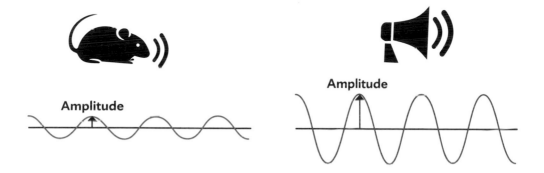

Low amplitude — Quiet sound

High amplitude — Loud sound

happens almost instantly, it involves a complex chain of events.

A sound's journey starts when the outer ear (pinna) gathers sound waves and directs them toward your eardrum, as shown in the illustration below.

Many mammals, like cats and dogs, can rotate their outer ears toward the source of a sound. But humans can't do this. Instead, sound waves reach your outer ears from different directions at different angles and at slightly different times and intensities, producing different patterns, depending on where the source of a sound is in relation to your head. This helps your brain to locate the source of the sound.

Using both ears to hear

The use of both ears is critical for locating the source of a sound. Hearing with two ears is called binaural hearing.

HOW HEARING WORKS

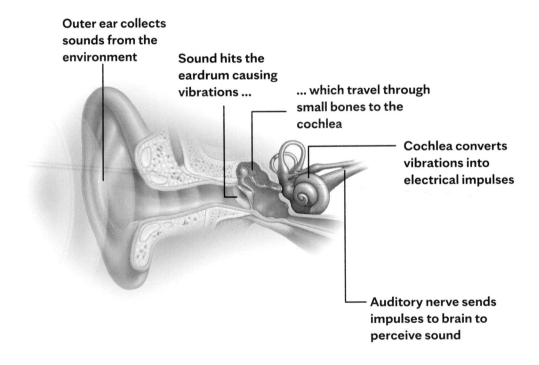

Outer ear collects sounds from the environment

Sound hits the eardrum causing vibrations ...

... which travel through small bones to the cochlea

Cochlea converts vibrations into electrical impulses

Auditory nerve sends impulses to brain to perceive sound

A sound occurring on your left will reach your left ear first and register as louder in this ear than in your right ear. When your brain compares information from both ears, it can distinguish whether the sound has come from your left or right.

With auditory information from both ears, your brain can often pick out the sounds you want to hear and somewhat suppress background noise. This is why you can hold a conversation with someone at a crowded, noisy party.

Into the middle ear

After a sound wave travels through the

SOUND PRESSURE LEVEL AND HEARING LEVEL

You're likely familiar with the term *decibel*. Decibels are common units of measure that can show two different types of sound intensity.

One type of sound intensity decibel is used to describe the sound pressure level. This is the force of a sound wave in the environment or the amount of pressure it exerts on your eardrum. A level of 0 decibels sound pressure level (dB SPL) is about the weakest sound that the best human ears can hear. To compare, the intensity of typical speech is generally around 60 dB SPL.

Decibels are also used to measure how well your hearing compares with the average for a large group of young people with typical hearing. This measure is expressed in decibels hearing level (dB HL).

When your hearing is tested, an audiologist may want to find out what your hearing threshold is. Hearing threshold refers to the faintest level at which you can perceive sound. People who are considered to have typical or near-typical hearing have a hearing threshold between 0 and 25 dB HL.

People who have trouble understanding conversations, on the other hand, may barely hear sounds at 40 dB HL but not lower. They're considered to have moderate hearing loss. Those who can hear only a loud, nearby voice may have a hearing threshold of 70 dB HL. These are people who are considered to have severe hearing loss.

In this book, sound intensity expressed in terms of dB represents a measure of sound pressure level. When referring to a measure of hearing level, it will be expressed as dB HL.

ear canal, it strikes the taut membrane of the eardrum, causing it to vibrate. These vibrations cause the ossicles that bridge the space between the eardrum and the oval window also to vibrate. The ossicles move together like a tiny lever system. See how this works on page 90.

Because the surface of the eardrum is much larger than the oval window, the vibrations are delivered with greater force to the inner ear. Sound waves create vibrations on the eardrum. The vibrations move the middle ear bones to send the sound waves to the oval window of the cochlea. The middle ear bones have to increase the intensity of the sound before it gets to the cochlea because sound waves do not travel as well through fluid as they do in the air.

Amplifying the sound increases the energy, which helps push the vibrations through the fluid of the inner ear. Because fluid poses more resistance than air does, it takes more force to push sound vibrations through it.

Into the inner ear

Once a sound wave passes through the middle ear, it reaches the cochlea in the inner ear. This snail-shaped structure is filled with fluid. Sound vibrations cause the fluid in the cochlea to ripple, causing a wave to continue to travel through the innermost parts of your ear.

Tiny sensors called hair cells ride this wave. They sense whether a sound is high-pitched or low-pitched. These hair cells also help send the sound wave toward the brain. During this process, chemicals that create an electrical signal are released, and the nerve from your ear (auditory nerve) carries the electrical signal to the brain. Once the signal reaches the brain, the brain turns the signal into a sound you can recognize.

Traveling to the brain

From the auditory nerve, electrical impulses travel to information-processing stations in the brain. These stations analyze the signals to figure out where they came from. They also filter out background noise.

In this process, signals from the ears are turned into sounds that you can recognize and understand. See a visualization of the sound pathways on page 93.

Scientists are still working to understand how the brain interprets the impulses and identifies them as distinct sounds. What they *do* know is that speech and language — how the brain gives meaning to sound — is associated closely with the ability to hear. Experts know that a person's ability to recognize and understand specific sounds starts early. For example, at about 3 months, babies can differentiate their parents' voices from other voices.

COMMON TYPES OF HEARING LOSS

With such a complex hearing system, even small changes or slight damage to the ear can affect your hearing.

IN THE EAR

Sound waves that have traveled through the ear canal cause the eardrum and ossicles of the middle ear to vibrate. These vibrations trigger a wave of fluid that bends the tiny hair cells in the cochlea causing a chemical reaction that sends electrical impulses along the auditory nerve and into the brain.

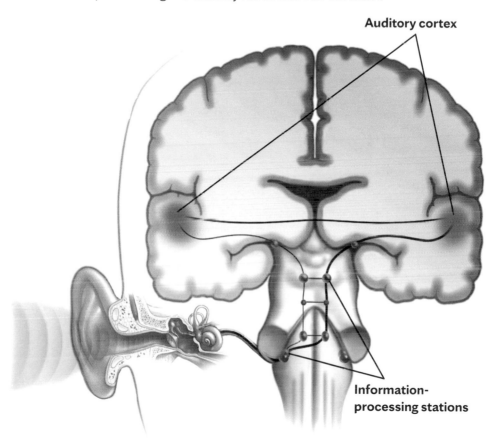

Auditory cortex

Information-processing stations

IN THE BRAIN

Electrical impulses from the auditory nerve pass through and cross between several information-processing stations on their way to the auditory cortex areas in the temporal lobes. There, the brain sorts, processes, analyzes, compares and files information about sounds, helping you to make sense of what you hear.

There are three types of hearing loss: conductive, sensorineural and mixed.

Conductive hearing loss

The ear canal and the middle ear conduct sound waves to the sensory receptors of your inner ear. If something blocks this pathway, the sound waves are disrupted. The result is a reduced perception of sound. This can occur from an excessive buildup of wax in the ear canal. Your ear canal usually cleanses itself, but in some cases buildup occurs and may require professional removal.

Other problems that can cause conductive hearing loss include foreign objects lodged in the ear, middle ear infections, head trauma and unusual bone growth in the region of the ear. Chapter 3 offers more information about conductive hearing loss.

Sensorineural hearing loss

Damage to the structures of the inner ear, like the hair cells in the cochlea or the nerve fibers leading from the cochlea to the brain, can cause sensorineural (sen-suh-ree-NOOR-ul) hearing loss.

People with sensorineural hearing loss often have trouble hearing sounds at high frequencies, like certain consonants used in speech. For example, someone with high-frequency hearing loss may not be able to tell the difference between the words *tell* and *sell* or *miff* and *myth*.

This damage is most often associated with the general wear and tear of aging, known as presbycusis (pres-bih-KU-sis), or with too much exposure to loud noise. Some diseases, certain powerful medications that can hurt the ear, physical trauma to the head and genetic disorders also can cause this type of hearing loss. Growths like tumors that damage the auditory nerve are another cause.

Although sensorineural hearing loss usually can't be reversed, hearing aids and other assistive devices and techniques can improve hearing enough to make effective communication possible.

Mixed hearing loss

Some people may have a combination of conductive and sensorineural hearing loss. For example, someone with age-related sensorineural hearing loss may also develop a middle ear infection. The

LEARN MORE

Get a one-minute summary of the main types of hearing loss and how they can be treated from Matthew L. Carlson, M.D., a Mayo Clinic ear surgeon: links.mayoclinic.org/hearingloss conductive hearing loss caused by the infection can usually be eliminated with medical treatment. However, the sensori-neural damage is likely untreatable.

How much hearing loss you experience from any of these types depends on a few key factors:

- **Cumulative noise.** A lifetime of hearing the sounds of power tools, machinery, firearms, appliances, concerts and motor vehicles can gradually affect your ability to hear.
- **Sudden intense noise.** A single loud noise from a nearby explosion or gunshot is another cause of sensorineu-ral hearing loss.
- **Medications.** Certain drugs are harm-ful to hearing (ototoxic). Their use can lead to permanent hearing damage.

COMPENSATING FOR HEARING LOSS

Overall, hearing helps you stay connected to the world. Losing some of your hearing can be an obstacle at best. Sometimes, it can be dangerous. While you may mostly credit hearing for helping you to under-stand what others are saying, it also cues you to where you are and alerts you to potential danger.

Many people avoid admitting to hearing loss. But acknowledging it is the first step toward re-engaging with the world around you.

Before you learn more in the following chapters, take a moment to assess your current hearing abilities.

Do you find yourself doing any of the following?

- Blaming others for mumbling or speaking too softly
- Limiting or avoiding social activities
- Turning up the volume on the television or radio
- Smiling and nodding without under-standing

If you answered yes to any of these, don't be afraid to ask for help. Consider talking to your doctor about your concerns and seeking the help of an audiologist. Ad-dressing a hearing problem can put you on the path to becoming a more active participant in life and a more engaged companion and friend.

Up next, you'll learn what happens when you bring your concerns to your doctor.

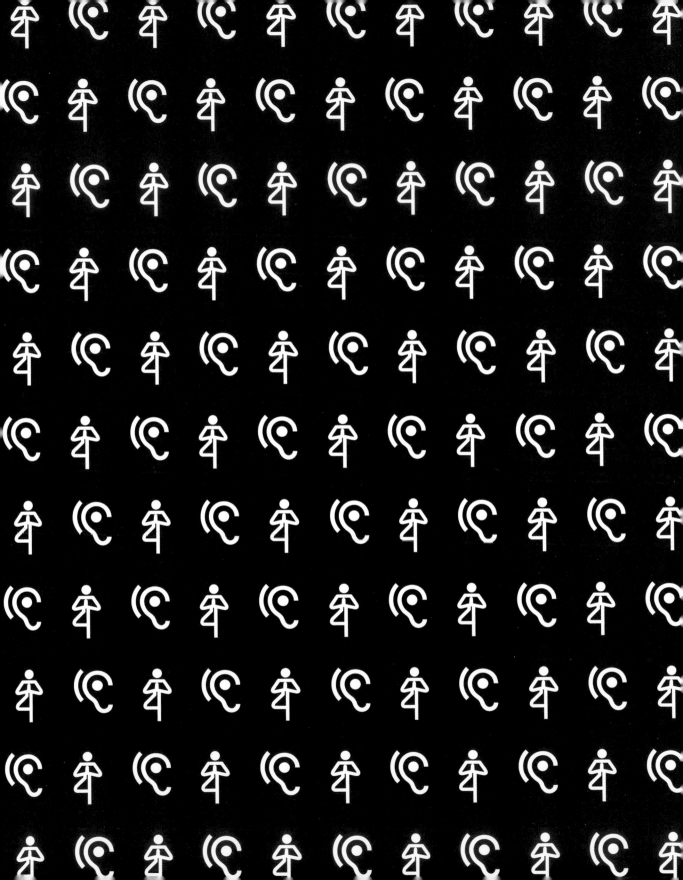

7

Getting a
hearing exam

Perhaps you've noticed lately that you have trouble hearing certain letter sounds when someone is talking to you. Or maybe while in a meeting, you've had difficulty hearing the speaker's voice over the background noise. Or you've been having trouble following typical daily conversations at the dinner table. Because you're unsure of what's being said, you've become more reluctant to join in conversations.

If these situations are becoming all too familiar, you may have some degree of hearing loss. While you may be tempted to just accept or ignore the problem, consider seeking help from a doctor.

A hearing exam may help identify what's causing your hearing loss. It may also lead to treatment that enables you to both

hear better and feel more socially engaged and confident.

Start the conversation with your primary doctor. A doctor may examine the ears and provide explanations for many of your concerns. A doctor can also refer you to a hearing specialist (audiologist) if needed.

In this chapter, you'll get a closer look at each of the specialists who may be involved in diagnosing and treating hearing loss. You'll also find out when a hearing exam may be needed, what happens during an exam, and what the results mean. Knowing what tests to expect and why they're done can help you get the most out of your hearing exam and put you on your way toward an effective solution.

WHO PROVIDES EAR CARE?

Your doctor may ask about your hearing at routine visits and encourage you to get your hearing tested if there are any concerns. Anytime you are routinely exposed to loud noise, notice signs of hearing loss, or notice a ringing, buzzing or roaring in your ears (tinnitus), your doctor is the best person to talk to.

Sometimes hearing loss is caused by earwax, an infection, a tumor or other problems that call for medication or surgery. That's why it's best to talk to your doctor about changes in your hearing — so you can get the appropriate treatment.

If you need more-specialized care, your doctor can refer you to a hearing specialist. Because hearing loss can have many causes, hearing specialists often work closely with other specialists to make a diagnosis and decide on treatment. Learn more about these specialists below.

Often, hearing specialists work together to diagnose and treat a condition. For

COMMON HEARING SPECIALISTS

If your doctor refers you to a hearing specialist, you may see one of these health professionals.

Otolaryngologist. This type of medical doctor is trained to diagnose and treat diseases of the ears, sinuses, mouth, throat, voice box (larynx), and other parts of the head and neck. An otolaryngologist may also do cosmetic and reconstructive surgery of the head and neck. This specialist is commonly called an ear, nose and throat (ENT) doctor.

Neuro-otologist. This kind of doctor specializes in physical problems of the ear, such as infections, facial paralysis, dizziness, hearing loss, ringing, buzzing or roaring in your ears (tinnitus), tumors and deformities of the ear that people were born with. If you need surgery for an ear disorder, you'll probably see a neuro-otologist or an otolaryngologist with special training in ear surgery.

Audiologist. A complaint of hearing loss without any physical signs of disease might result in an appointment with an audiologist. An audiologist can assess and determine the severity of hearing loss and also help with hearing aids and hearing rehabilitation when needed.

Because some drugs can damage hearing, an audiologist also may monitor the hearing of people who are receiving treatment for an illness, such as cancer or an infectious disease.

example, a neuro-otologist or an ear, nose and throat specialist (otolaryngologist) may refer you to an audiologist to have your hearing tested before treating an ear disorder, and again later to see if the treatment is working.

Or if an audiologist thinks a medical problem is causing your hearing loss, you may see a neuro-otologist or an ear, nose and throat specialist for treatment. After treatment, you may see the audiologist again for hearing rehabilitation. Which specialist you see and when is important. That's because each specialist approaches a problem with different training and from a different perspective.

SCHEDULE FOR HEARING EXAMS

It's important for everyone at every age to get hearing tests. If you're concerned about hearing loss or you've been in a situation that increases your risk of hearing loss, you can ask for a hearing exam. Sometimes, a hearing exam is required by law.

Screening for newborns and children is done regularly (see Chapter 12). Screening for adults, on the other hand, is done only when it's needed. The American Speech-Language-Hearing Association recommends that adults get their hearing checked at least every 10 years through age 50 and every three years after that.

Screening is especially important in midlife and later because hearing loss increases with age. Just 2% of adults ages 45 to 54 have hearing loss. But in adults ages 55 to 64, this number increases to almost 1 in 10. About 1 in 3 people between the ages of 65 and 74 and nearly half of the adults older than age 75 have hearing loss.

Where you work also factors into how often you need to get your hearing checked. Continuous exposure to loud noise can cause you to lose your hearing little by little over time — and this hearing loss can be permanent.

To help prevent work-related hearing loss, the Occupational Safety and Health Administration (OSHA) requires employers to monitor noise levels if they're 85 decibels (dB) or higher on average over eight working hours. If workplace noise reaches this level, the employer must develop and maintain a hearing conservation program at no cost to the employee.

The program must include record keeping, free regular hearing exams, noise monitoring, and access to earplugs or protective devices like earmuffs. The employer must also provide employees with training on hearing protection. OSHA requires that a qualified hearing specialist administer the program.

If regular screening shows that hearing loss has occurred, the employee must be told about it and wear hearing protectors in work environments with noise levels of 85 dB or more. Hearing protectors are required for all employees when noise levels exceed 90 dB, averaged over eight working hours. Hearing protectors have to fit properly and be worn continuously during periods of noise exposure.

TYPICAL HEARING EXAM

If you have concerns about hearing loss, it's best to bring them up to your doctor. From there, your doctor may refer you for additional lab tests or to an audiologist.

An audiologist usually assesses all aspects of hearing. Your hearing history will likely be taken, and your ears will likely be examined. You may have lab tests. You'll also typically have hearing-specific tests, including audiometry, speech reception and word recognition. You'll learn about these tests in detail next.

If it looks like you have hearing loss, the doctor or audiologist will usually evaluate your signs and symptoms and see if other medical conditions may be causing the hearing loss. The exam will also help show how severe the hearing loss is and what treatment would help most. Here's more on each part of a typical exam.

Medical evaluation

A full medical evaluation is the first part of a hearing exam. It offers a snapshot of your overall health and helps show if your hearing loss could be the result of an underlying condition.

Before your exam, be prepared to answer questions like these:
- When did you first become aware of the signs and symptoms of hearing loss?
- Is your hearing loss affecting one ear or both ears?
- Is your hearing loss getting worse, improving or staying the same?
- Are some sounds more difficult to hear than other sounds, or are all sounds equally hard to hear?
- Do you have trouble recognizing where a sound comes from?
- Do you have ear pain, discharge, infection, dizziness, ringing in the ears or loss of balance?
- Does anyone in your family have hearing problems?

Be sure to mention if you've had long exposure to loud noise or any head trauma, ear surgery, or chronic illness. Also mention if you've recently had an upper respiratory infection, like a cold or pneumonia. What medications you take or have taken is also important to share.

Physical exam

Next, you'll have the size, shape and position of your outer ear (pinna) inspected for swelling, deformity or redness.

You may also have your eyes, nasal cavity, mouth and neck checked for any problems that might be associated with ear damage. A slender, flexible tube with a light at the end is used to check for signs of fluid buildup or infection in the back of your nose and upper throat (nasopharynx) and your eustachian tubes, which connect your ears to your nasopharynx.

Otoscopy

The visual examination of the ear canal, eardrum and middle ear is called an otoscopy. The prefix oto- means "ear." For the test, the doctor or audiologist will likely use an otoscope (see below). Its light and magnifying lens make it easier to see inside the ear. A special microscope called an otomicroscope also may be used to view the ear canal and eardrum.

Generally, this exam is painless and takes just a minute or two. It helps show earwax, fluid buildup, foreign objects, a tumor or skin irregularities in the ear canal, and any small tears in the eardrum.

Otoscopy also shows the color of your eardrum — whether it is clear and has its usual pearly gray color. If your eardrum membrane is bulging, this may mean you have fluid in the middle ear.

GETTING AN OTOSCOPY

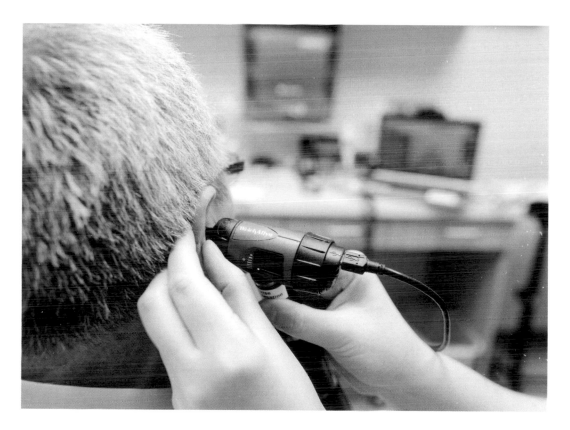

During an otoscopy, a doctor or an audiologist uses an otoscope — an instrument with a light and magnifying lens — to see inside the ear.

Tuning fork test

A tuning fork looks like a dining fork with only two tines. Made of steel, it sounds a single tone when struck against a solid object — and that tone varies according to the shape and thickness of the tines.

For this test, vibrating forks with different pitches are placed near the ear. They measure hearing sensitivity to the air conduction of sound waves. The forks are also placed against the skull to measure sensitivity to the bone conduction of sound waves.

Comparing the results of these tests provides important clues to the cause of the hearing loss. Some people hear better when the tuning fork is placed against the skull. That means a loss of hearing may be because of a conductive hearing loss,

EAR INFECTION

This illustration shows what the inside of the ear looks like when it's infected.

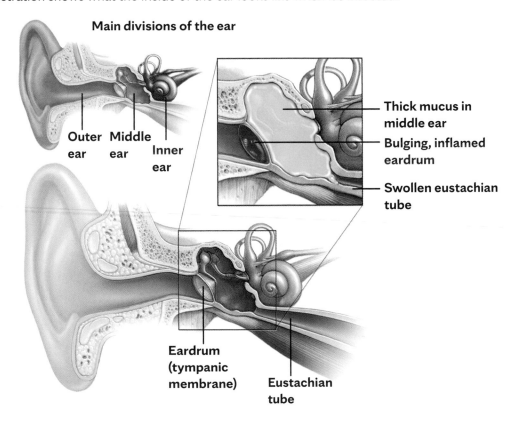

Main divisions of the ear

Outer ear Middle ear Inner ear

Thick mucus in middle ear

Bulging, inflamed eardrum

Swollen eustachian tube

Eardrum (tympanic membrane)

Eustachian tube

meaning that sound waves are having trouble passing through the ear canal or middle ear. If there's no difference in hearing ability with the tuning fork near the ear or against the skull, the hearing loss is likely caused by damage in the inner ear.

Lab tests

You may have a blood test to confirm or rule out infectious or inflammatory diseases linked to hearing loss. Syphilis, German measles (rubella), cytomegalovirus (CMV) and several autoimmune disorders are all examples.

Blood tests are particularly important for pregnant women. Any one of these diseases in expectant mothers can lead to hearing loss in babies when the babies are born. Blood samples also may be examined for DNA irregularities.

Imaging tests

If it's possible that a tumor, tissue irregularity or damage to the auditory nerve is causing your hearing loss, you may have imaging tests like an MRI or CT scan.

MRI creates detailed images of soft tissues using magnetic fields and radio waves. A CT scan produces images of bone structure from a series of X-rays. Both tests can reveal disorders that would otherwise remain unseen. Other imaging tests may be used to locate irregularities you were born with (congenital) and trauma to the ear.

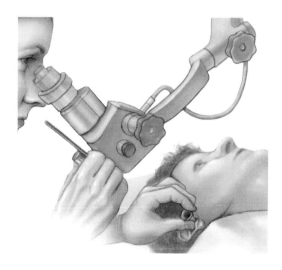

An otomicroscope provides a more detailed look into the ear. A small viewing funnel is gently inserted into the ear canal to focus the image.

EAR FILLED WITH WAX

This illustration shows what the inside of the ear looks like when it's full of wax.

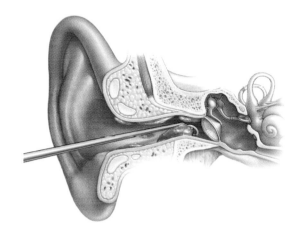

Audiological evaluation

This series of tests focuses on how well you hear. Audiologists use several tests to determine your hearing status and degree of hearing loss.

These tests show differences between types of possible hearing loss. They also reveal whether hearing loss is affecting one or both ears. In addition, these tests show if the hearing loss involves one, two or more frequencies. Repeat testing can show if the impairment is getting worse.

Audiometry

This testing measures your ability to hear pure tones. The tuning fork test you read about earlier is a simple form of audiometry. There are two types of testing: air conduction and bone conduction.

To check your hearing by way of air conduction, you'll have earphones placed over your ears or small, soft tips placed into your ear canals. Tones are played through the earphones to one ear at a time. The frequency and intensity of the tones will vary.

When you hear a tone, you'll be directed to signal, usually by raising a hand or pressing a button. Your responses are recorded on a type of graph called an audiogram. This test shows the faintest sounds you can hear, known as your hearing thresholds.

To check how well you hear when sound waves are passed through the bones of your skull, you'll have a vibrating device placed either behind your ear or on your forehead. Sound vibrations travel through your skull and directly stimulate your hearing organ (cochlea). This testing bypasses any blockage that may be present in the outer ear or middle ear.

If test results show that you hear sound when it's conducted through skull bone better than through the ear canal and middle ear, then sound isn't getting through the outer ear and middle ear properly. This means you probably have some form of conductive hearing loss. If results show that your hearing is no better via bone conduction than through air conduction, you likely have a problem in your inner ear (sensorineural).

Speech reception test

For this test, the audiologist plays a recording of, or speaks, familiar two-syllable words, like *pancake* or *baseball*, while you listen through headphones.

As you hear a word, you repeat it or point to a picture of it. The intensity of each word gradually softens. The faintest level of speech you can understand at least half the time is called your speech reception threshold (speech recognition threshold, or SRT).

If your SRT is typical — usually between 0 and 25 decibel hearing level (dB HL) — it generally shouldn't be hard for you to hear, and you should be able to understand conversational speech in a quiet environment. An SRT that's 26 dB HL or

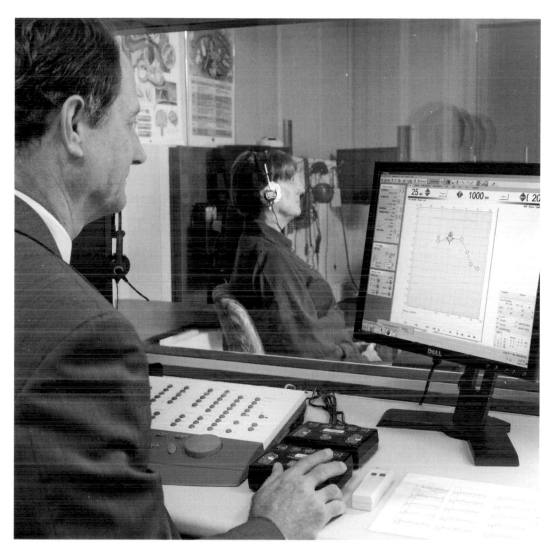

During audiometry, you'll sit in a sound-treated room (top). The audiologist is usually in a separate room. You'll signal whenever you hear a tone played through the earphones. How well you hear different pitches will be recorded on an audiogram (bottom). The audiogram also charts other hearing-related qualities.

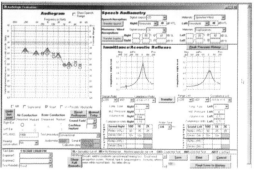

higher points to more-severe levels of hearing loss. An SRT that's higher than 91 dB HL means profound hearing loss. Generally, the SRT and audiometry test results match up.

Word recognition test

This test determines how well you can understand speech at a comfortable volume. It's also known as a speech discrimination test.

You'll be asked to identify a series of familiar single-syllable words, like *come*, *thin*, *sack* and *knees*. When you hear the words, you repeat each word or point to a picture of it. Occasionally, background noise is added to see how distraction affects your understanding.

Your score reflects how many words you've identified correctly. This score helps the audiologist understand how much difficulty you may have understanding conversation in a quiet environment and whether this is expected for your level of hearing loss.

When it's done with and without a hearing aid, a word recognition test may suggest how helpful a device is for you and whether it makes sense to use one.

Other tests

In addition to a medical exam and an audiological exam, you may have other aspects of your hearing tested. These tests can help refine your diagnosis or point you toward the best course of treatment. Here's more on some of the additional tests you may have.

Tympanometry

This test checks how well the eardrum and middle ear work. Tympanometry (tim-puh-NOM-uh-tree) helps detect conditions like a perforated eardrum, fluid in the middle ear and reduced air pressure in the middle ear that causes the eardrum to suck inward (retract).

For this test, a soft probe is placed in the ear canal. As small, varying amounts of air pressure are directed toward the ear, the probe measures the eardrum's movements. The results are charted on a graph called a tympanogram.

On a tympanogram, a typical response shows a line rising to a sharp peak in the middle of the graph, like a mountain peak. If you have fluid in the middle ear, the eardrum won't move easily, and the graph's line won't peak. The graph can also show a pressure difference in the middle ear that happens when you feel as if your ear needs to pop.

Acoustic reflex test

An acoustic reflex test measures the level at which the muscle in the middle ear contracts in response to loud sounds.

First, some background: The acoustic reflex protects the inner ear from sounds that are too loud. This reflex doesn't mean that your ears will always be protected from damage that can happen from a loud sound, however. That's because there's a slight delay between the auditory nerve's response to a sudden sound and the middle ear muscle's protective contraction. This brief delay leaves the inner ear vulnerable to damage from impact noise. Because of this delay, a nearby gunshot, for example, may cause immediate, permanent damage to the ear.

During an acoustic reflex test, you'll hear sounds at varying levels of intensity. The sound level that causes your middle ear to contract — or if your middle ear *doesn't* contract in response to sound — provides information about your hearing loss.

LEVELS OF HEARING LOSS

Decibel (dB) range	Level of hearing loss	Characteristics
16 to 25 dB HL * **	Slight	• Has difficulty hearing faint or distant sounds
26 to 40 dB HL	Mild	• Occasionally misses consonants • Has increasing difficulty in understanding speech with noisy backgrounds and faraway speakers
41 to 55 dB HL	Moderate	• Can understand regular conversation if face to face and vocabulary is controlled
56 to 70 dB HL	Moderately severe	• May miss most of what's said in a regular conversation • Has trouble hearing in a group setting
71 to 90 dB HL	Severe	• May not be able to hear speech unless very loud • Needs amplification to be able to take part in a conversation
91 dB HL and above	Profound	• May not be able to hear speech at all • Relies on visual cues such as lip reading or sign language

* dB HL = decibels hearing level
** Most clinics consider 0 to 25 dB HL to be the range of standard hearing sensitivity.

Based on American Speech-Language-Hearing Association, 2013

Auditory brainstem response test

This test measures the electrical nerve impulses sent from the inner ear to the brain when sounds are introduced to the ear. It shows how well the inner ear, called the cochlea, and the brain pathways for hearing are working.

Electrodes are placed around the ear and on your head. Earphones introduce a series of short clicking sounds to your ear. A computer connected to the electrodes records the activity that happens when the auditory nerve sends the impulses to the brain.

Because this test doesn't require a response — with a hand signal, for example — it's often used with newborns and infants. It can also assess other problems with the auditory nerve. It's also used for adults with hearing loss that's more severe in one ear than the other.

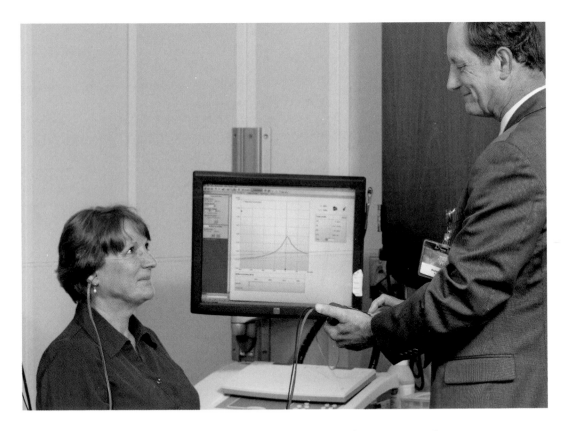

Your doctor or audiologist may use tympanometry to see how your eardrum responds to varying amounts of air pressure. The tympanogram can show whether your hearing problems are linked to an outer ear or inner ear (conductive) issue, like a perforated eardrum or fluid buildup in the middle ear.

Otoacoustic emissions test

This test measures how the hair cells of the inner ear respond to the movement of fluid in the cochlea.

When your hair cells vibrate, they produce sounds called otoacoustic emissions. You can't hear these sounds, but a probe equipped with a microphone, placed in the ear canal, can measure them. This test is useful because people with typical hearing produce otoacoustic emissions, but people with hearing loss caused by damaged hair cells don't.

Results from this test help show how severe hearing loss is. This test is also used to screen hearing in newborns and infants because it doesn't require a voluntary response, like the raising of a hand in response to a tone. This test is also useful for people receiving certain medications that can damage hearing.

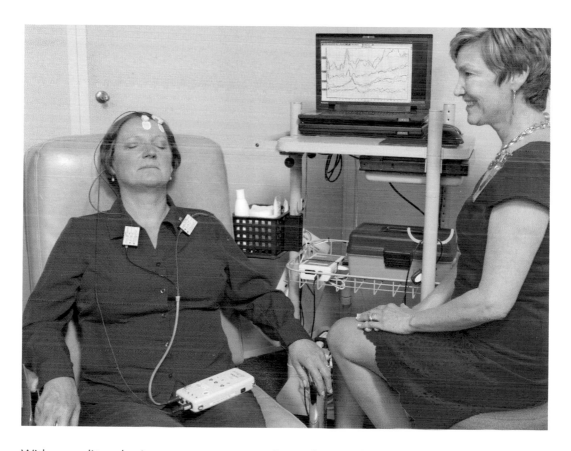

With an auditory brainstem response test, electrodes attached to the ears and head measure how the auditory nerve receives electrical impulses from the inner ear and transmits them to the brain.

UNDERSTANDING YOUR AUDIOGRAM

Any or all of the tests you've learned about in this chapter may be used to compile a detailed assessment of your hearing. This assessment is known as an audiogram.

An audiogram is a graph that reveals the softest sounds you can hear at different pitches. An audiogram portrays sound in terms of two of its most important qualities: pitch (frequency) measured in hertz (Hz), and loudness (intensity) measured in decibels (dB).

See an example of an audiogram on the next page. Across the top of the box, you'll see a range of frequencies, from a low (bass) pitch on the left (125 Hz) to a high (treble) pitch on the right (8,000 Hz). For reference, the frequencies most common in human speech are between 500 Hz and 4,000 Hz.

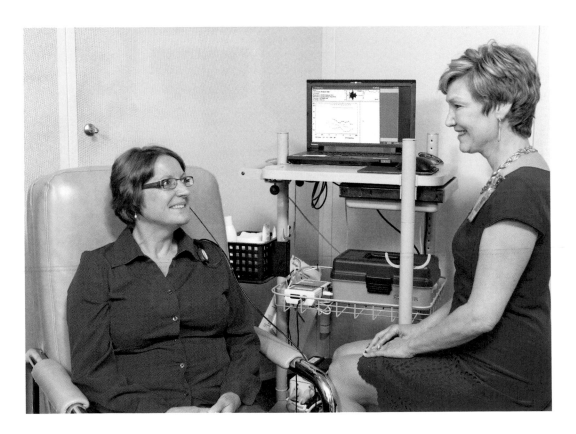

During otoacoustic emissions testing, a probe with a small microphone is placed in the ear canal. This microphone checks for inaudible sounds called otoacoustic emissions. These emissions are produced in people with typical hearing, but not in people with hearing loss.

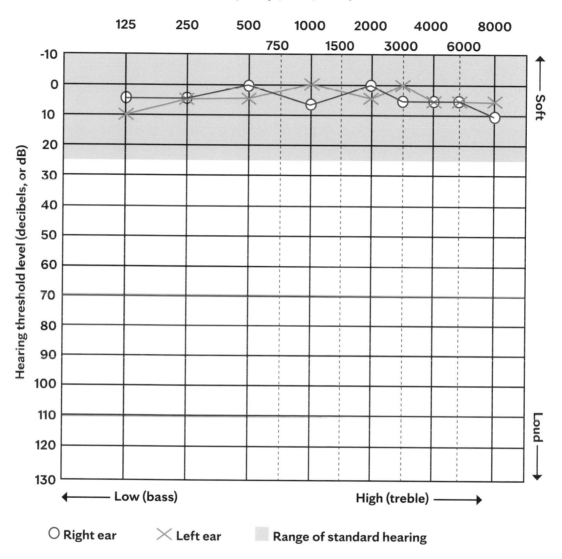

Frequency (hertz, or Hz)

O Right ear   ✕ Left ear   ▨ Range of standard hearing

This audiogram shows regular hearing in both the right ear and the left ear. Hearing in the right ear is plotted with O's and in the left ear with X's. If you have typical hearing, all your X's and O's will typically fall in the range between minus 10 and 25 decibel hearing level (dB HL) — the shaded area on the audiogram. As hearing loss develops, the X's and O's fall lower and lower on the graph, and below the shaded area.

THE SPEECH SPECTRUM

The banana-shaped area of speech represents all of the sounds that are part of conversational speech. If you have mild or moderate hearing loss, you likely can't hear certain sounds. If you have severe or profound hearing loss, you likely can't hear conversational speech sounds unless they are made louder by hearing aids.

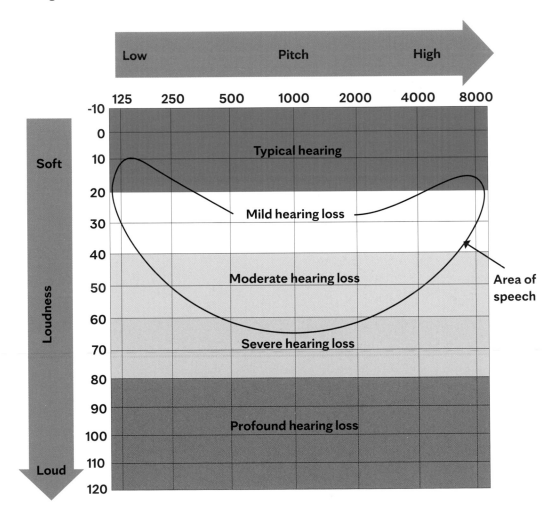

Based on the American Speech-Language-Hearing Association, 2021

The horizontal lines on the audiogram represent how loud the sound is. Zero dB HL represents very faint sounds that someone with typical hearing can generally hear.

Every point on an audiogram represents a different sound, determined by its pitch at a given intensity.

While an audiogram provides a number of details related to hearing, pure tone audiometry (page 104) is the test used most to assess hearing loss.

THE SPEECH SPECTRUM

If your audiogram represented all of the sounds that make up human speech at a typical conversational level, it would show up as a banana-shaped area just above the middle of the graph. This area, shown on page 112, is known as the speech spectrum. Soft, high-pitched sounds like *ss*, *ff* and *th* would be in the right part of the spectrum. Loud, low-pitched sounds like *zz*, *j* and *n* would appear in the left part. Sounds like *ch* and *g* fall somewhere in between.

If you placed an image of the spectrum over results from your audiometry test, you would be able to see which parts of conversational speech are easy for you to hear and which ones aren't. The sounds that you can't hear can be heard only if the decibel level is increased and the sounds are louder.

Hearing loss is generally greater in the high frequencies. This is where many of the consonant sounds occur. Often, people who can't hear in these frequencies say they can hear speech, but they can't understand it.

WHY HEARING EXAMS ARE IMPORTANT

Sometimes you don't think about getting your hearing checked until you notice that something is obviously wrong or another person notices and calls attention to the hearing problem.

Protecting your hearing can have an immediate and positive physical, social and emotional impact on your life. Treatment may help eliminate feelings of isolation and frustration and allow you to participate more actively in the world around you. A decision to take action today and schedule a hearing exam can determine how well you'll be hearing in the weeks, months and years ahead.

PART 4

Living well with hearing loss

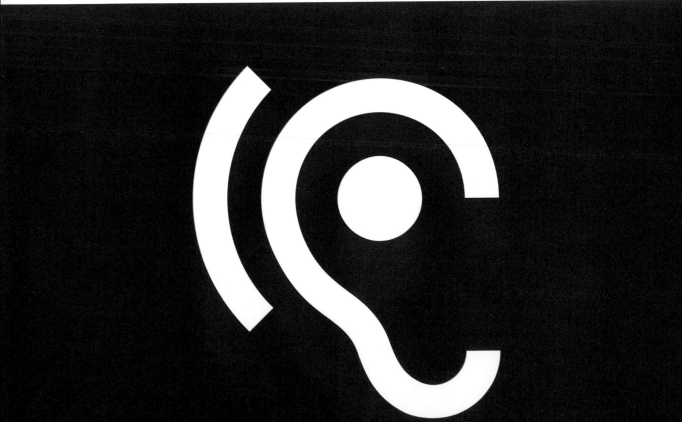

8

Quality of life

When Ken was a Navy midshipman, his left ear was damaged during a gunnery practice. Although his right ear worked hard to make up for what he couldn't hear with his left ear, Ken still faced challenges. Making sure his "good" ear was near the person talking to him and sitting at the front of the room in meetings were a way of life. Although Ken got by and felt like he was coping well with his hearing loss, the daily obstacles he encountered were sometimes hard to overcome.

Like Ken, Julie was often rushing to the front of the room for presentations so that she could clearly hear the speaker. Diagnosed with bilateral sensorineural hearing loss when she was in her 20s, Julie pursued a career in teaching but eventually resigned when she felt she was no longer being fair to her students.

Ken's and Julie's experiences illustrate the fact that hearing loss means more than just losing one of your senses. It may also mean missing out on cherished experiences and the activities you enjoy. If you have hearing loss, you may feel excluded and stop trying to interact with others or the world around you.

For all these reasons and more, hearing loss can significantly impact quality of life.

By taking steps to improve their hearing, both Ken and Julie regained the things in life that they enjoy — and you can, too. Use their experiences, which you'll read about later in this chapter, and the practical advice on the following pages and in the next two chapters to guide and encourage you.

Sound helps anchor you to the world around you. Sound gives you pleasure and a sense of belonging. Sound also alerts you to danger or opportunity.

Hearing impairment may deprive you of these experiences. You may not be able to listen to the laughter and conversation between friends at a social gathering or the inspiring sounds of nature on a forest trail. Activities like eating at a restaurant; traveling; attending religious services, classes or concerts; and watching movies become more difficult. This was the case with Ken, who could navigate many situations well despite his hearing loss — except for times when he was in a restaurant with friends and there was

ARE YOU PUTTING OFF GETTING HELP?

If you're having trouble even thinking about talking to your doctor about your hearing loss, you're not alone. Many people deny that they're having trouble hearing and put off a visit to the doctor.

Here are a few reasons why:

It's so gradual, you don't notice it. Hearing loss usually develops over time, so you may not recognize the problem at first. Without even realizing it, you may have found ways to compensate for your hearing loss. For example, maybe you've gotten good at reading people's lips without realizing it.

You're hearing people just fine — you just don't always understand them. Many people underestimate the severity of their hearing loss. When people lose their hearing, they tend to lose the ability to hear high-pitched tones first, like consonant sounds. Consonants are the sounds of speech that provide clarity and crispness to what you hear. So when you experience hearing loss, voices may still sound loud, but they also seem unclear.

You don't want people to think you're old or incapable. Many people are concerned they'll be stigmatized just by wearing a hearing aid. A common concern expressed by people coming to terms with hearing loss is that others might assume they're also losing the ability to think and act independently.

The truth is, hearing loss is more common than you might realize — and there's no shame in coming to terms with it and taking steps to make your situation better. The sooner you seek help to improve your hearing, the more quickly you can get back to all the things about your life that make it worth living.

background noise and several people were speaking at the same time. Even something as routine as talking on the phone, shopping for groceries and running errands can pose challenges.

Frequently, hearing loss happens little by little over several years. For that reason, it may take time to recognize that you're having trouble hearing. In fact, family and friends may notice your hearing loss before you do.

Initially you may deny or try to minimize the hearing impairment, perhaps because you can still hear certain sounds well. This was Ken's experience. "I was in denial, not willing to spend thousands of dollars on my hearing when I thought I was coping. I was satisfied with the friends I had, the work I was doing. Life was good," Ken said. You may even convince yourself that if other people spoke more clearly or slowly, you'd be able to hear them just fine.

Denying your hearing difficulties won't make them go away. On the contrary, muddling through life with hearing loss may only create more issues. Instead, look honestly at your life. Take stock of the areas where hearing loss is causing problems, and see what adjustments you can make to improve your experiences. Use the suggestions in this chapter to guide you.

ADDRESSING COMMON CHALLENGES

People with hearing loss often face similar challenges. Feeling disconnected from others is usually at the top of the list, both at home and at work. Access to information also is affected. Hearing loss may also impact your sense of identity. In turn, these struggles may cause you to feel anxious or depressed.

Relationship obstacles

Humans are social creatures — most people seek out connections with others and thrive on them. Living in an intensely social world can be difficult when your ability to communicate is hampered. Hearing loss can strain your relationships with family, friends, co-workers and anyone with whom you interact regularly.

For example, when you can't hear much of what's being said at a dinner party, you may tire quickly or feel left out. This may cause you to skip these events and stay home. At the store, you may have trouble hearing your charge total from a soft-spoken cashier. If your spouse calls to you while you're working in front of a running faucet or dishwasher, you may not understand the words. Other factors associated with hearing loss, like social isolation, low self-esteem and depression, may further strain relationships.

When you struggle to hear, conversations can quickly become frustrating and tiresome. Although you want to spend time with your family and friends, interacting may get too stressful. It's natural to try to avoid situations that you know will be difficult. In so doing, you may cut yourself off from the world around you and the people who love you.

Research shows that people with hearing loss who don't use hearing aids are more likely to withdraw socially and become depressed.

By contrast, older adults with hearing loss who use hearing aids or other devices tend to have a higher quality of life, better relationships with their families and better feelings about themselves. They are more socially active, experience more interpersonal warmth and have greater emotional stability.

To minimize the negative effects of hearing loss, it's important to remain socially involved. Chats with friends, attendance at family gatherings, dinner parties and card games, and evenings at the movies or theater — these pleasurable activities keep you involved in the mainstream of life.

Find strategies to improve communication and social interaction — both for yourself and for people involved in your day-to-day life — starting on page 120.

Loss of identity

Hearing loss affects how you perceive your place in the world. Many adults whose hearing loss occurred early in life have, over time, incorporated the impairment into their self-image. It's a part of who they are. As a result, they're more used to managing hearing loss in their daily lives and routinely cope with it. But for adults who lose hearing later in life,

EMOTIONAL SIDE EFFECTS OF HEARING LOSS

If you've been living with hearing loss for any amount of time, it probably won't surprise you that researchers have uncovered links between hearing impairment and depression and anxiety. If you can't hear well, you may avoid being around other people. This self-imposed isolation may lead to loneliness, which in turn, leads to depression.

A similar cycle can happen with anxiety. Not being able to hear the world around you may cause you to feel anxious. Then if you avoid being around others because it makes you feel anxious, you may become withdrawn and depressed.

Getting treatment for hearing loss can break this cycle. Some research shows that using hearing aids improves both social function and symptoms of depression. But above all, know that your feelings are real, and they're legitimate. Give yourself a break, feel what you're feeling, and then take the steps you need to so that you can keep moving forward.

the impairment can be more disruptive. They may worry about what others think of them, concerned that they'll be seen as incompetent. They often feel inadequate, and this affects their daily activities.

As you take steps to address your hearing loss, keep in mind first and foremost that hearing loss doesn't diminish your value. You still have much to offer this world. By addressing your hearing loss, you'll be better equipped to continue living a life of meaning and value.

Workplace issues

For many people, a large part of meaning and value comes from work. Hearing impairment can cause challenges in the workplace if you misunderstand a conversation with your manager or supervisor because of background noise in the office or shop. It may be difficult to hear someone speaking to you through a glass partition, like a bank teller's window, or from another room. You may have trouble taking part in meetings or conferences when several people are talking quickly all at once.

Despite these obstacles, hearing loss doesn't have to put an end to your work life. Practical solutions to many common workplace problems are available.

First, it's useful to know your legal rights. Almost every state has a statute making it illegal to discriminate in employment on the basis of disability, race, religion, sex, age or other minority status. Under the Americans with Disabilities Act (ADA), it's against the law to discriminate against qualified people with disabilities in job application procedures, hiring, firing, advancement, compensation and training. Find information about these regulations at the Department of Justice website (*www.ada.gov*).

In addition, the ADA requires employers to make what's called reasonable accommodation for employees with disabilities, including hearing loss. A reasonable accommodation can be any adjustment to a work environment that enables the employee with a disability to perform essential functions of the job.

For employees with more-severe hearing loss, reasonable accommodations may include providing a teletypewriter (TTY) or telecommunications device for the deaf (TDD), captioned telephone, videophone or even something as simple as a flashing ringer on the regular telephone.

Sound barriers or muffling can be added to office walls and floors to control background noise in the work environment. Assistive listening systems can be installed in auditoriums and meeting rooms. The services of a transcriber or sign language interpreter can be sought out. In addition, employers should change or add lighting to make it easier to see.

State governments also offer programs aimed to help people with disabilities keep their current jobs or, if that's not possible, retrain for other jobs. Certified counselors in these programs are trained to help people with disabilities by addressing work-related concerns.

Adjusting in the workplace

While there are steps your employer can take to create a more accessible workplace, you can also take steps to enhance your environment. Try these tips.

Use communication aids. Assistive listening devices like telephone amplifiers, FM systems, captioning and alerting devices are all examples. You'll learn more about these resources in Chapter 11.

Limit background noise. If you can, locate your desk so that it isn't near busy hallways and noisy office machines, such as photocopiers, and air conditioners.

Ask co-workers to address you by name as they speak. This allows you to focus your attention, understand what's being said and participate in discussions.

Sit up front at meetings and presentations. Arrive early or ask to sit close to the speaker.

Give yourself a break. Try to schedule time for breaks between situations that require a lot of listening and communication. This can help prevent fatigue.

Alert your co-workers. If you know of situations that may cause problems, talk to your co-workers about them. Let them know how they can help.

IMPROVING SOCIAL INTERACTION

Many strategies can help you communicate well and stay involved in activities.

Effective communication can occur even if you don't hear each and every sound. Your remaining hearing, along with visual information, context clues and life experience, helps you understand speech. With the assistance of technology, the impact of hearing loss can be considerably reduced.

Here are several techniques that can enhance your interactions with others.

Speak up when you need to

Let others know your needs. If you don't speak up for yourself, you may not hear or understand anything in a conversation.

Be direct about what it takes for you to participate and interact with others. These strategies can make a difference:

- Let others know that you have hearing loss. Then they won't think you're aloof or forgetful.
- Keep in mind that your hearing loss affects other people, and be prepared to deal with their reactions.
- Be willing to use hearing aids and assistive listening devices.
- Ask for, but not demand, help when you need it.
- Tell people exactly what you need. You may ask individuals to slow their speech, look at you when they speak, move a hand away from their face or repeat a phrase.
- Take a break from conversation when you're tired.
- Show your appreciation when others make an effort to communicate better with you.

- If you're taking your emotions out on others, be willing to admit it.
- Modify your environment to fit your hearing needs.

When you're direct with others, you'll likely find it easier to cope with many social situations. Most people are willing to help if you tell them you're having trouble hearing.

Create an environment for better listening

One of the most effective strategies for better hearing and social interaction is to modify situations that make listening difficult. Often, by altering your environment, you can prevent communication breakdowns. These suggestions can help:

Move closer to the source of the sound you want to hear

Examples include a television or stereo system, a public speaker or lecturer, or a visitor to your home. Arrange your home or office furniture so guests or family members are seated nearby and facing you directly. If you can't organize the arrangements, choose your own seating so that you're close enough to see and hear the person you want to engage with.

Move away from distracting or overpowering noise

When you're in public places, don't sit close to machinery, appliances or busy hallways. In a restaurant, request a table away from the kitchen, lobby, bar or other noisy spot, and sit with your back to the wall. Don't sit close to music speakers or ventilation ducts.

At home, turn off or mute the television or radio when you're talking with someone. Sit away from open windows that let in traffic noise and outdoor sounds.

Position yourself so that the speaker's face is visible and well lit

Visual cues like facial expressions or the position of a speaker's head may provide clear indications of what's being said. Good lighting helps with speech reading, which you'll learn about shortly.

Plan in advance for social activities

Before attending an event in a busy or crowded setting, call ahead to see if the facility uses assistive listening devices. Arrive early to pick up the devices and so that you have a choice of seats.

Learn speech reading

Speech reading, also called lip reading, is a tool that people with hearing loss can use in many social situations. With this technique, you learn to recognize spoken words by watching the movements of the speaker's lips, tongue, lower jaw, eyes and eyebrows, as well as facial expressions, body stances and gestures. These visual cues are critical for understanding the words being said.

Most people, whether they hear well or not, rely on speech reading to some degree. In fact, many are unaware that they can speech read. For example, when background noise is extremely loud, people with typical hearing may try instinctively to match the motion of the speaker's lips to the sounds they hear.

COMMUNICATING WITH SOMEONE WHO HAS HEARING LOSS

When you're conversing with someone who has hearing loss, keep in mind that what to you is simple communication may be a tiring effort for your companion. A person with hearing loss has to make an active effort to understand. Hearing aids may help, but turning up the volume won't make distorted sounds any clearer.

Enhance communication with someone who has hearing loss by using these practical suggestions:

- Before starting to talk, reduce the level of background noise. Turn off the television, radio, air conditioner or other noisy appliances. Don't leave a faucet running. If you can't reduce background noise, try to move to a quieter area.
- Make sure you have the person's attention before speaking. You can do this by saying his or her name or touching his or her shoulder.
- Talk face-to-face. Speak at eye level, no more than a few feet away. Don't chew gum, smoke, talk behind a newspaper or cover your mouth while you're having the conversation.
- Speak at a typical conversational level, especially if the person is wearing hearing aids or has a cochlear implant. Don't shout. If necessary, modestly increase your volume.
- Speak clearly but naturally. Slow your speech a little, using a few more pauses than usual.
- Use facial expressions, gestures and other body language cues to make your points.
- Watch your listener's face for signs that comprehension is a problem. Rephrase your statements if the listener is unsure of what's been said.
- Alert your listener to changes in topics of conversation.
- Show extra consideration in a group situation. What's known as cross-talk is one of the most difficult situations for someone with hearing loss. Try to structure events so that only one person is speaking at a time. At meetings, it's helpful to display an agenda on a board or monitor and, as the meeting progresses, to indicate which item is under discussion.

Speech reading works best if you still have some hearing ability left and use hearing aids or other assistive devices. It's accomplished mainly by following lip patterns — the shapes made by people's mouths when they speak. For example, the vowel o is formed with rounded lips, the consonant m is made by pressing the lips firmly together, and the consonant l requires placing the tongue behind your teeth.

But even the most skilled speech reader can't pick up every word. Not all sounds can be seen on the lips, and some sounds look exactly alike. For example, the consonants b, m and p look similar on the lips. So the words ban, man and pan are almost impossible to tell apart.

Other factors — rapid speech, poor pronunciation, bad lighting, averted face, covered mouth, facial hair — can make speech reading more difficult. You often need to rely on the context of the sentence and other nonverbal cues to understand what's being said.

As with any new skill, learning the basics for speech reading takes time and patience. For people with hearing loss, including those with hearing aids, speech sounds may be muted or distorted. Speech reading requires you to focus on the lip movements.

But your skill usually improves with practice, and the more you practice, the more confident you'll become. Many proficient speech readers find that this technique allows them to follow conversations more easily. In fact, some people who are profoundly deaf choose to communicate using speech reading and speech rather than sign language.

Tips for speech reading

Rather than trying to catch every word that's spoken, focus on the overall intent and context. Here are other suggestions for making speech reading easier:

- Position yourself so that a light source is behind you and you can clearly see the speaker's face. If you can't see the speaker's face well, you won't be as able to speech read.
- Identify the topic being discussed as quickly as possible. If you are familiar with the topic and can identify key words, you won't need to analyze every phrase.
- Watch the speaker's facial expressions, body language and gestures for clues.
- Before you enter a conversation, inform the person who's speaking that you have hearing loss. Encourage the person to speak at his or her regular speed, but maybe a little slower.
- Try to relax as much as possible. Don't try to understand everything. This can make speech reading that much more difficult.
- Use your remaining hearing alongside speech reading. Diminish background noise by turning off the television or radio, closing the door or window, or sitting in a quieter section of a restaurant, away from the bustle.
- Focus on the message rather than specific lip movements. You'll find that subsequent sentences may clarify the words you've missed.

- If you can't fill in a missing word, ask the speaker to rephrase the sentence in a different way.
- Take frequent breaks, especially when you're first learning to speech read. The technique requires deep concentration, and you may tire quickly from the effort. When you get the chance, close your eyes and relax for a few minutes.

Use sign language

Sign language uses hand signs — made with hand shape, position and movement — as well as body movements, gestures, facial expressions and other visual cues to form words. It's often the first language of many people who are deaf or have severe hearing impairment. Sign language is a complete language with distinct grammar, semantics and syntax.

Different sign languages are used in different countries and regions of the world. American Sign Language (ASL) is commonly used in the United States and Canada. Like the English language, ASL allows for regional differences and jargon.

Sight is considered the most valuable tool for using sign language. Each sign in this language may be broken down into parts in the same way that spoken words can be broken down into individual sounds and intonations. Each ASL sign is a combination of hand shape, hand movement and hand location. Changing any one of these parts changes the meaning of the sign.

Facial expressions and body movements also are important in sign language. For example, English speakers usually use a raised tone of voice to signal that they're asking a question. ASL users ask a question by raising their eyebrows and widening their eyes. Stating a command may require them to sign more emphatically.

Using sign language takes time and practice, and learning from a book is difficult. Enrolling in classes and meeting with other people who use sign language is generally recommended. Picking up enough signs for basic communication can take a year or more of training.

Community colleges, universities, libraries, continuing education programs and vocational rehabilitation centers are some of the institutions that may offer sign language classes. The American Sign Language Teachers Association (ASLTA) certifies qualified teachers. The ASLTA website (*www.aslta.org*) has information about state and local chapters.

Consider a hearing dog

You're probably familiar with guide dogs for people who are blind. Did you know that service dogs are also available to help people with severe or profound hearing loss? Hearing dogs can alert you to everyday sounds such as a doorbell, ringing telephone, oven timer, alarm clock, and smoke and fire alarms. A dog can even respond when someone calls your name.

Hearing dogs don't bark to get your attention. Rather, they're trained to use their noses or paws to nudge you, then

KEN'S STORY: 'I HARDLY EVER MISS A WORD'

Until a few years ago, Ken's quality of life wasn't as good as it could be. His phone conversations were short, and dinners with friends were a struggle. This all changed when he started using rechargeable hearing aids with a remote microphone that he can use with Bluetooth devices, like his smartphone. You'll learn about these technologies in Chapter 11.

Although Ken has been using hearing aids for many years, recent advances in hearing aid technology have dramatically improved his quality of life.

"The connection with the smartphone has made all the difference," Ken says.

When Ken's smartphone rings, he pushes the button on his microphone to answer, which connects the call directly to his hearing aids. The remote microphone also allows Ken to have clear conversations with someone in another room, and to hear someone speaking to him easily even if they're in a group or a restaurant with background noise. If Ken's in a meeting, he can set his remote microphone in the middle of a table near the person speaking and get every word. This means Ken no longer has to race to the front of a room to grab a good seat just so he can hear.

Ken's friends, who remember how short their phone calls used to be, have noticed the change. "They say, 'You're more willing to talk longer with your new hearing aids,'" Ken says. "There isn't the struggle to hear or decipher conversation anymore. With the mic set on Bluetooth, I can talk to people on the phone and I hardly ever miss a word."

Newer hearing aid technology also helps Ken enjoy traveling from his home in the Midwest to warmer climates when the snow flies. His trek takes him through a number of states, where he stops to catch up with friends. Dining in restaurants, visiting art museums, and taking tours along the way are all part of the experience — and with newer hearing aid technology, Ken can enjoy all of these excursions thoroughly.

For Ken, hearing aid technology helps him participate in all of the things in life that bring him meaning and joy.

"Life is for living the best way you are able," Ken says.

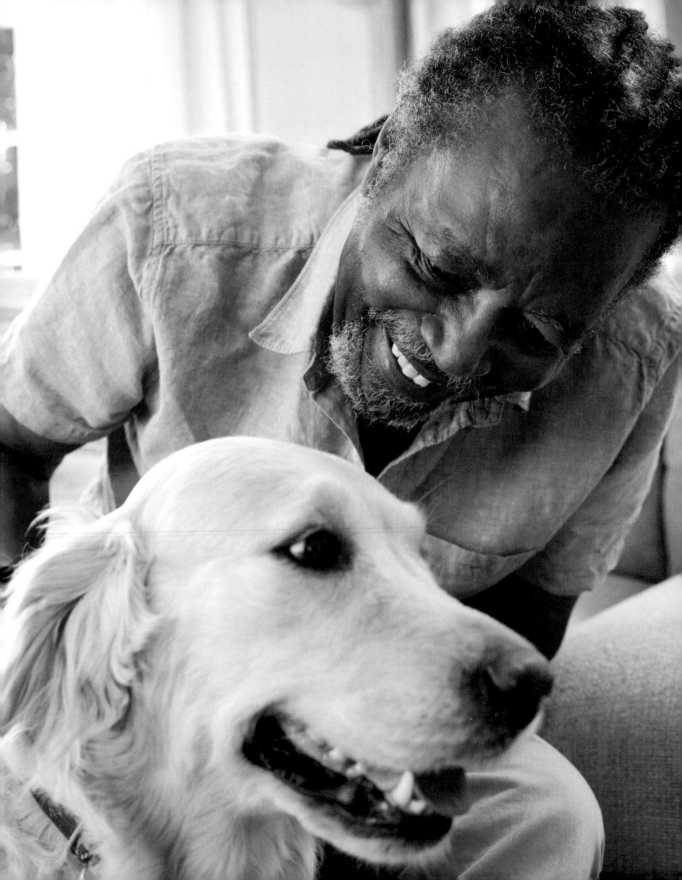

lead you to the source of the sound. Hearing dogs can also carry messages or notes between you and another household member.

Paying attention to your hearing dog's reactions in public spaces can help you be more aware of car traffic and pedestrians, especially when they approach you from behind or around a corner.

According to the Americans with Disabilities Act, hearing dogs must be allowed to accompany their owners into businesses and other places that serve the public. Often a bright orange or yellow leash identifies a hearing dog. But the dog doesn't have to have special identification to accompany you into a business or public space.

Hearing dogs come in all shapes and sizes. Many are taken from animal shelters and given several months of training — obedience training as well as special service training. There's no national training standard, and the dogs aren't required to be certified, though many are.

Some people with hearing loss choose to participate in the training, working

WORKING TO IMPROVE LACK OF ACCESS

Have you ever strained to understand what's being said over a public address system? Have you found yourself not able to enjoy the theater because you can't hear the actors unless they speak in your direction? Have you struggled with schoolwork because the classroom either mutes or echoes the teacher's voice? Situations like these can be stressful for anyone in an active life. They present unique challenges for people with hearing impairment.

All too often, people with hearing impairment don't have the communication tools they need for travel, entertainment, education and medical care. Few movie theaters provide captioning services or assistive listening systems. Many medical clinics and hospitals don't have interpreters on staff.

Organizations like the Hearing Loss Association of America (HLAA) are working to improve access in a variety of situations for people with hearing loss. Improvements in assistive technology are allowing more people with hearing loss to participate in a greater range of activities. The advent of online learning has improved access to education.

For more information about assistive listening devices, captioning and other communication aids, see Chapter 11.

directly with a private trainer and the dog. Others prefer to get a dog that's already trained. Regardless, you may have to wait two or more years before getting a canine companion.

In the United States, two well-known hearing dog organizations are Paws With a Cause and Canine Companions for Independence. Most service dog organizations are nonprofits that provide dogs at no charge to people who need them.

FIND SUPPORT

In this chapter and throughout this book, one message is constant: You are not alone in your hearing loss. Many people live — and live well — with hearing impairment, and you can, too. In addition to the tips you've learned about so far, these additional sources of support can help you adjust to life with a hearing impairment.

Hearing rehabilitation

If you don't feel comfortable with your hearing impairment, consider hearing rehabilitation, also called aural rehabilitation or auditory training. Hearing rehabilitation helps you adjust to hearing loss and tries to reduce the difficulties. Advocates say that by making the best use of hearing aids and assistive listening devices, you can take charge of your communication needs.

An audiologist, a speech-language pathologist or both typically provide hearing rehabilitation services. You may work one-on-one with a therapist or as part of a group or in both settings. Group therapy can be especially helpful because you'll meet others facing the same issues as you are.

The overall goal of hearing rehabilitation is to maximize your self-confidence and your ability to communicate with others in everyday situations. This can be achieved by:

- Understanding your hearing loss
- Learning how to listen
- Learning skills in speech reading
- Building confidence in communication situations
- Dealing with emotional problems related to hearing loss
- Learning about all the options among different hearing aids and assistive listening devices
- Understanding your legal rights and being your own advocate
- Promoting your family's understanding of your needs
- Making it easier for your family to communicate with you

You may attend rehabilitation sessions at a medical clinic, rehabilitation center, community college or private office. Software programs can be used at home and at your own pace of learning. Your hearing health care provider can discuss these programs with you.

Support groups

Sharing experiences with other people with hearing impairments is a great way

JULIE'S STORY: 'I FEEL BLESSED'

When Julie was diagnosed with mild hearing loss in her 20s, she was told she would be deaf by age 40. She knew no one else her age with hearing loss. Hopeless and alone, Julie saw no reason to consider hearing aids.

Julie's friends got frustrated when she misunderstood things, shied away from talking on the phone or didn't want to go out. Eventually, Julie said, "This outgoing person became reclusive."

All of this changed one day, about 10 years later, when a friend convinced Julie to attend a college class with him. As it turned out, the class was filled with audiology students eager to talk to people with hearing loss. The students' gentle encouragement and budding expertise gave Julie the support she so desperately needed. Through this experience, Julie was encouraged to consider hearing aids.

It took Julie another year just to decide to get fitted with hearing aids. But eventually, after she started using hearing aids regularly, Julie's quality of life began to improve.

Julie credits some of the biggest changes to her quality of life with hearing impairment to finding others she could relate to. She did this in large part by getting involved with the Hearing Loss Association of America. Through her involvement with the organization — she started its first chapter in Wisconsin — Julie learned about technologies she didn't know existed. And she did so alongside hundreds of others she could relate to — people with hearing loss who wanted to get back to truly living life.

"We learned so much from each other. And we learned, first, that we were not alone," Julie said.

Eventually, Julie earned her master's degree and returned to teaching, the profession she loved and left behind after she was diagnosed with hearing loss. "I feel blessed to have been able to learn about technology that gave me my life back," Julie said.

to find support. Belonging to a group can remind you that you're not alone in dealing with this problem.

Support groups aren't the same as group aural rehabilitation. An audiologist leads an aural rehabilitation group. Peers frequently lead support groups. Support groups are an excellent resource for problem-solving and mutual support. They're also a way to meet potential new friends. How have others handled traveling, meetings, telephone conversations, communicating in public places or dealing with difficult work colleagues? What problems have they had with hearing aids? Have they used assistive listening systems?

Many national organizations with local chapters provide support groups for people with hearing loss. These include the Alexander Graham Bell Association for the Deaf and Hard of Hearing, the Association of Late-Deafened Adults, the National Association of the Deaf, the Center for Hearing and Communication, and the Hearing Loss Association of America (HLAA). See "Additional resources" at the back of this book for contact information for these organizations.

National, state and local resources

Dozens of national, state and local organizations provide services for people who are deaf or have hearing loss. Resources include advocacy, education, financial aid, referral, advice on medical issues and counseling on work-related issues.

There are also opportunities for self-help and support groups, recreational and

SEEK OUT INFORMATION

You can find hundreds of products, publications, services and websites devoted to hearing impairment. But be careful. The information ranges from solid research to outright quackery.

When evaluating information you find online, consider these guidelines:
- Look for websites created by national organizations, universities, government agencies or major medical centers.
- Search for the most recent information you can find.
- Check for the information source. Notice whether articles refer to published research. Look for a board of qualified professionals who review the content before it's published. Be wary of commercial sites or personal testimonials that push a single point of view.
- Double-check the information. Visit several sites and compare the information offered.

social activities, and spiritual needs. Most organizations have websites and publications about hearing loss that offer easy-to-understand information.

The federal government provides information on affirmative action programs, reasonable accommodation and improving accessibility for people with disabilities. For example, if you feel your legal rights have been violated, you may contact the Equal Employment Opportunity Commission for advice, either by phone (800-669-4000) or on the web (*www.eeoc.gov*).

States provide services for individuals who have hearing loss, including vocational rehabilitation programs for people with disabilities. Offices that provide rehabilitation services often provide counseling and job retraining and may help pay for hearing aids.

Some states have programs to provide amplified telephones to people with hearing impairment. A state human rights or human relations commission or a governor's committee on employment of people with disabilities can provide information on related laws.

LIVE WELL WITH THE RIGHT TOOLS

Hearing loss affects many areas of life, including family, relationships and your social life. With the right support and tools, you can overcome any challenges you face and live well with hearing loss.

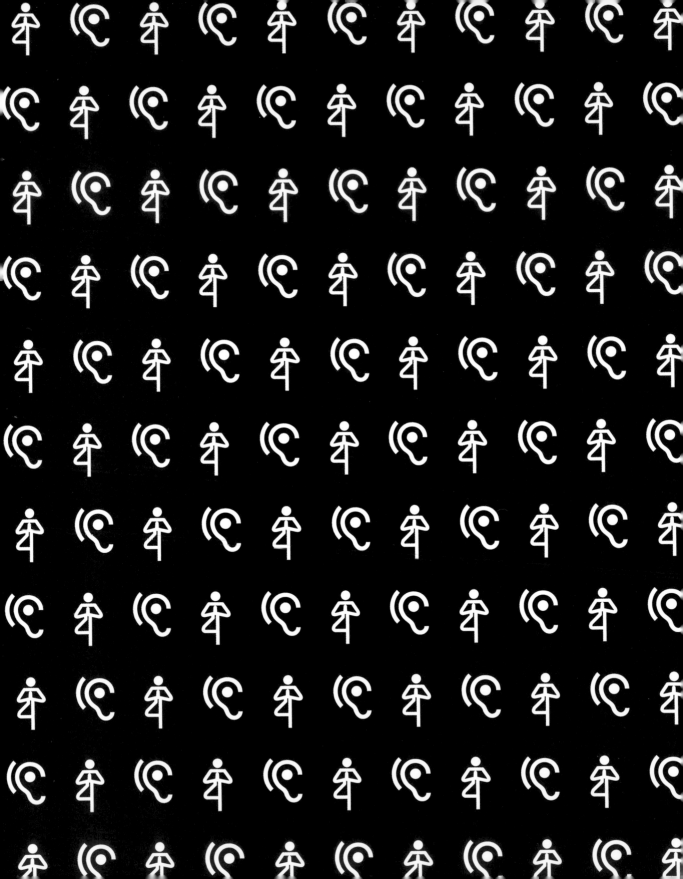

CHAPTER | 9

Hearing aids

"I don't think it's any less intimidating today for someone who doesn't want to wear a hearing aid than it was for me when I got my first one," says Julie, as she reflects on being diagnosed with hearing loss in her 20s and getting her first hearing aid. You read about Julie's hearing loss experience in Chapter 8.

"I didn't want to wear it. I was sure it wouldn't help me. It cost too much. Yet, I had reached a point where I was desperate. I was slowly leaving the hearing world where I had grown up, become educated and worked," Julie says. "Looking back, I am so thankful for all the technology I have benefited from."

Hearing loss doesn't mean you're cut off from the world of sound. But it does mean that you may need a little help hear-ing sounds and understanding them. If you feel like you're missing out on life because of hearing loss, chances are that you'll benefit from a hearing aid, like Julie has. Hearing aids are the single most effective treatment for most people with hearing loss.

Hearing aids are sophisticated electronic devices that make sounds louder. They don't restore hearing to what it was, but they can help you hear better and communicate in daily activities.

Hearing aids can enhance personal interactions. They assist with many problems linked to hearing loss, like trouble understanding conversations and being aware of signals, timers and alarms. Hearing aids can help with feelings of isolation and problems with self-image.

Hearing aids have improved tremendously in recent decades. Years ago, hearing aids were large and clunky. Their sound quality was poor — harsh and distorted like that of a cheap transistor radio. The sound quality they offer is much better today than it once was. Many options are available to match different lifestyle and communication needs.

Hearing aids are also much less visible than older models. As you read through this chapter, take a look at the photos and guess which people are wearing hearing aids and which ones aren't. Find the answer at the end of this chapter.

Adjusting to a hearing aid takes some time, but you'll start to enjoy your improved ability to hear and communicate in a variety of social situations. When you wear your hearing aid regularly and take good care of it, you'll likely notice improvements in your quality of life.

This chapter outlines how hearing aids work and how to choose the one that might work well for you.

Motivation is the key to success with hearing aids. People who are committed to the process and have a positive attitude usually have the best outcomes. They're also more apt to continue wearing the devices and gain the most benefit.

There are a variety of hearing aid styles. Hearing aid styles are often based on specific needs. Each person and each type of hearing loss is different. Before making a selection, it helps to be informed, patient, and open to the suggestions that an audiologist or hearing aid specialist offers.

QUESTIONS TO ASK YOURSELF

Before meeting with your audiologist or hearing aid dispenser, give some thought to these questions.

How challenging is it for you to:
• Talk with one or more people in a noisy environment?
• Watch television without having to turn the volume way up?
• Hear and recognize someone who calls you on your telephone?
• Hear your phone ring from another room?
• Hear someone ring your doorbell or knock on your door?
• Hear traffic?
• Feel confident and included in social settings?

Knowing what challenges you experience helps your audiologist or hearing aid dispenser find the right hearing aid for you.

WHAT'S IMPORTANT TO YOU?

Selecting a hearing aid depends on what's important for you. Think about when communication is the hardest for you. When is it important for you to hear well? Are there times when you're exhausted by having to focus so hard on hearing? Maybe you want to hear your children or grandchildren when they visit, or to understand conversations during a weekly card game.

Take a moment to write down the answers to these questions:
- What situations are challenging? When and where do you face the biggest challenges?

- What makes these situations difficult? Be as specific as you can.

- How did these situations make you feel? Did you let your family or friends know that you were having trouble?

There are several ways to increase hearing aid satisfaction. You've probably already taken the first steps — acknowledging your hearing loss, having your hearing tested and looking into solutions to the challenges you're facing. Simply acknowledging your hearing loss and seeking help is a strong sign that you'll have success with a hearing aid.

Learning about your specific type of hearing loss also is helpful. This can help with developing realistic expectations about what hearing aid might work best for you. Everyone experiences varying degrees of success with hearing aids.

How well hearing aids function depends on many things, including the type of hearing loss and how severe it is. If you expect a hearing aid to restore perfect hearing, you're bound to be disappointed. That's why it's important to know what you can realistically expect from a hearing aid.

Next, think about your goals and hopes. What motivates you to *want* to wear a hearing aid? How much does the style of the device matter to you? What extra options are important? Choosing the device that's right for you depends on your specific needs.

HEARING AID MARKET IS GROWING

About 1 in 10 Americans has some degree of hearing loss. Here's how many of them wear hearing aids:
- Age 65 and older — Just over 41%
- Ages 35 to 64 — Almost 23%
- Age 34 and younger — About 30%

All told, less than half the people who could benefit from using a hearing aid actually wear one.

While these numbers haven't changed much over the years, research shows that around the world, the hearing aid market is growing and will continue to expand in the next several years as populations age.

Market analysts think this increase is partly due to the fact that hearing loss is becoming more common. In addition, people are generally more aware of the advancements being made in hearing aids, many of which you'll read about in this book. Hearing aids are also more available than they've been in years past. Slowly, hearing aids are becoming more accepted among those who can benefit from them.

All the components of this in-the-ear style of hearing aid are held in a small plastic container called the shell or casing. In a behind-the-ear style of hearing aid (see page 143), the casing rests behind the ear and the amplified sound is sent through a tube to the ear or an electrical signal is sent through a wire to a speaker that sits in the ear.

Microphone

The microphone picks up sounds, converts them into electrical energy (signals) and delivers them to the amplifier. This aid has one microphone. Some aids have two microphones, allowing you to pick up the sounds directly in front of you more than those coming from other directions and in noisy environments.

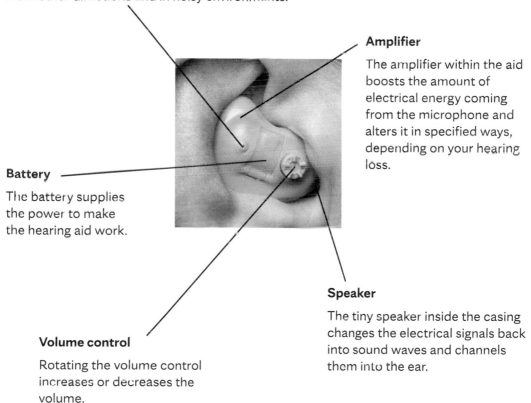

Amplifier

The amplifier within the aid boosts the amount of electrical energy coming from the microphone and alters it in specified ways, depending on your hearing loss.

Battery

The battery supplies the power to make the hearing aid work.

Speaker

The tiny speaker inside the casing changes the electrical signals back into sound waves and channels them into the ear.

Volume control

Rotating the volume control increases or decreases the volume.

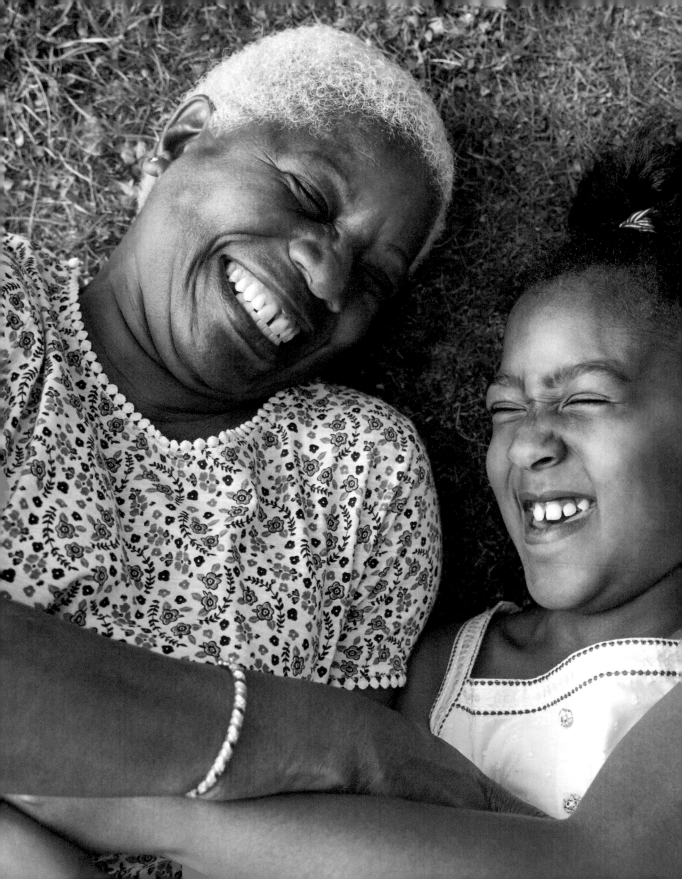

When you think about the type of hearing aid to buy, keep in mind that there will likely be trade-offs among many factors. Performance, style, size, technology and cost are all examples. For instance, you may want the smallest device available. Or maybe you want a hearing aid that's easy to operate, regardless of size. Think about what's most important to you and what trade-offs you're willing to accept. If you're retired and spend most of your time at home, for example, you may not need the most expensive model with all the latest bells and whistles.

Consider talking to others with hearing loss who wear hearing aids. You already heard from Julie at the start of this chapter and Ken in Chapter 8; you'll read Greta's story later on in this chapter. And of course, talk to your audiologist and other hearing specialists. They'll be the ones working with you through the process of choosing, getting fitted for and adjusting to life with a hearing aid. Talking through expectations with these specialists helps ensure the best results.

HOW HEARING AIDS WORK

There are many types of hearing aids available, and technology is improving every day. But the purpose of all hearing aids is the same: to make sounds loud enough for you to hear them.

Hearing aids collect sounds from the environment via a small microphone. The sounds are then amplified and directed into the user's ear via a speaker. The amplified signal stimulates the inner ear,

ARE TWO HEARING AIDS BETTER THAN ONE?

Can you hear better with a hearing aid in each ear? In most cases, the answer is yes. Wearing two hearing aids has many advantages over wearing one. With two hearing aids, more sound information is sent to your brain. Plus, the signals reaching each ear differ slightly. This makes it easier to hear speech in situations where there's background noise.

With two hearing aids, you also experience more balanced hearing, at a volume that's more equal in both ears. Having two ears to listen with helps you locate the origin of sounds more easily, so you won't have to turn your head around to figure out who's talking. Another advantage of wearing two aids is that neither device needs to be turned up as loudly as when you're wearing only one. This helps reduce feedback and increases comfort.

Cost and not being able to wear a hearing aid in one ear may keep some people from wearing two hearing aids. Talk to your audiologist about your options.

activating nerve fibers that carry the sound impulses to the brain.

The illustration on page 137 labels the parts of what's known as an in-the-ear style of hearing aid. Its basic parts are found in all hearing aid styles.

With hearing aids, you're typically able to understand a conversation without needing to strain as much. They generally make it easier to hear people talking in a soft voice. You'll probably be able to turn down the volume of your television to a level that's more comfortable for others in the room who don't have hearing loss. Hearing aids can also help you hear environmental sounds, which gives you a better sense of what's taking place around you.

Hearing aids may help in situations in which it's hard to hear, like a theater performance or worship service when the speaker is far away or the sound is weak. They can help you feel more at ease when you're on your own — for example, while shopping — or when someone isn't talking directly to you.

Although hearing aids help improve hearing, they won't provide a completely natural sound. Hearing aids are electronic devices that make sound louder, based on your hearing loss. The new sounds that come through the hearing aids probably won't sound like what you're used to hearing. They'll have a different quality. Plus, hearing loss can cause the ear to distort some sounds. Hearing aids can't eliminate this distortion, so some sounds may not be crystal clear. While you may

notice that many things sound a little different when you first listen through a hearing aid, you'll likely adapt to this change quickly.

Finally, you may continue to have problems understanding speech in certain situations. For example, when there's background noise or many people talking at once, hearing aids can't isolate the voice that you want to hear from other sounds. Remember that even with typical hearing, background noise often affects understanding. However, some newer hearing aids have features that may help you in challenging listening situations. Learn about these features in Chapter 11.

HEARING AID STYLES

The type of hearing loss and how severe it is helps guide you toward the hearing aid that's best for you. For most people, traditional hearing aids and hearing devices that work through bone conduction are the main two choices.

Traditional hearing aids

Traditional hearing aids take sounds, make them louder and channel them into the ear canal (air conduction). This allows for better processing inside the ear.

These hearing aids come in many styles. They differ in size and in how they fit in the ear. Some are small enough to fit deeply in the ear canal. This makes them almost invisible. But the most widely sold aids are those that fit behind the ear.

With so many styles to choose from, keep in mind that the choice of a hearing aid depends on much more than just looks. The style that suits you best depends largely on your hearing test results. With that said, in general, the smaller the hearing aid, the less powerful it is and the shorter its battery life. If you hear well at low frequencies but not as well at higher frequencies, this also is a factor in what hearing aid may work best.

The size and shape of the outer ear, especially the ear canal, also may eliminate certain styles. For example, in-the-canal styles can be hard to fit in smaller ears. And if you have trouble manipulating small objects, a small hearing aid may not work well. Some medical conditions, like ear drainage, poor ear formation and hearing loss that's getting worse over time also may dictate which hearing aid style is best.

Here's more on the main types of traditional hearing aids.

Completely in the canal

The smallest hearing aid commonly available is called a completely-in-the-canal (CIC) aid. All parts, including the battery, are in a tiny shell or casing that fits deep inside the ear canal. A thin, plastic pull cord on the aid sticks out into the bowl-shaped part of the ear to help in removal. This type of hearing aid is used for mild to moderate hearing loss. If the ear canal is small or unusually shaped, this type of hearing aid may not be an option. It's not used in children or infants.

Hearing aid manufacturers are developing progressively smaller versions of CIC aids. This style may be referred to as a mini CIC, micro CIC or an invisible-in-the-ear (IIC) hearing aid.

Advantages The CIC aid is the least visible hearing aid. It may help reduce problems with wind noise. You can hold a phone over your ear as you usually would with this hearing aid.

Disadvantages The CIC style may not be as powerful as other types of hearing aids, so it may not be suited for severe hearing loss. CIC aids also have less space for options like volume control or directional microphones.

In addition, the batteries are small, so battery life is shorter. They're susceptible to problems with earwax clogging the speaker and microphone openings. Finally, the proximity of the microphone to the speaker may cause feedback.

In the canal

An in-the-canal (ITC) hearing aid fits partly in the ear canal but not as deeply as a CIC aid. The outer edge of the aid extends into the bowl of the ear. ITC aids can accommodate mild to moderately severe hearing loss, but they're not for use with infants and children.

Advantages ITC aids are designed to be discreet. They'll likely be more powerful than a CIC aid, with more opportunity for add-on features. You can hold a phone over your ear as you usually would.

Disadvantages Like CIC aids, ITC aids can be difficult to handle and insert into the ear. Some users may also find them difficult when replacing batteries.

In the ear

An in-the-ear (ITE) hearing aid fits into the bowl-shaped area of the outer ear. It comes in one of two options: a full-shell style, which fills most of the bowl-shaped area of the ear, or a half-shell style, which fills the bottom part of the bowl-shaped area of the ear. Low-profile is another option; it fills the bowl-shaped area of the ear but has a shallower fit. ITE aids are suitable for mild to severe hearing loss.

Advantages ITE aids can be more powerful than smaller aids, and they can accommodate more options, like a telecoil and directional microphones (for more on options, see pages 149-154). They're appropriate for a wider range of hearing loss. The battery may be larger and easier to insert than are batteries for the in-the-canal styles. You can hold a phone over your ear as you usually would. In addition, rechargeable batteries are available for ITE hearing aids.

Disadvantages ITE aids may pick up more wind noise than the smaller in-the-canal styles do.

Behind the ear

Behind-the-ear (BTE) hearing aids have two parts. A small plastic casing that rests behind the ear contains the hearing aid circuitry: the microphone, amplifier and speaker. The casing is often connected to a custom-made ear mold (earpiece) by plastic tubing. The tubing may be standard, thin or slim. The earpiece directs amplified sound into the ear canal. BTE aids can be used for almost all types of hearing loss, no matter how severe it is, and for people of all ages.

BTE aids are often mistakenly seen as old-fashioned and not technologically advanced. But in fact, BTE aids use the latest digital technology and may offer the greatest improvement in hearing, especially for more severe hearing loss.

Advantages These are the most powerful hearing aids available, and they can be programmed for any level of hearing loss. There's also plenty of space for options. BTE aids are the best style for infants, children and people with severe hearing loss. BTE aids are also the easiest to take care of, partly because changing the battery is easier when compared with other styles. BTE aids also usually need fewer repairs than other styles do.

Disadvantages Some people simply don't have enough space between their ear and the side of their head to make a BTE aid work. Also, this style may pick up more wind noise than the smaller aids do. You may have to hold a phone close to the microphone at top of your ear.

Receiver in the canal or receiver in the ear

Receiver-in-the-canal (RIC) or receiver-in-the-ear (RITE) hearing aids typically have

HEARING AID STYLES AT A GLANCE

This side-by-side comparison offers a closer look at the main styles of hearing aids.

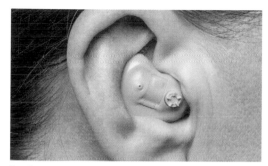

In the ear

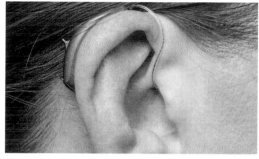

Receiver in the canal

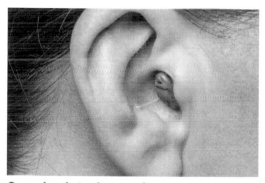

Completely in the canal

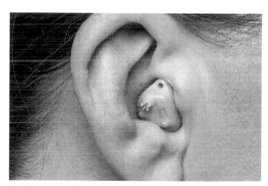

In the canal

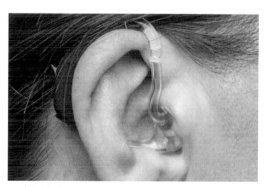

Behind the ear

a small casing that fits behind the ear and houses the microphone and amplifier. The casing is connected by a tiny wire to the speaker that sits in the ear canal. The speaker can be fitted into the ear canal with a custom ear mold or a soft, flexible dome-shaped tip.

Advantages This type of hearing aid is small and less obvious. This can make it more cosmetically appealing. Because the receiver is close to the eardrum, feedback is less of an issue than it is with open-fit BTE aids. The speaker can be replaced in the office, avoiding a factory repair.

Disadvantages RIC and RITE receivers can be susceptible to earwax. In addition, smaller aids use a small battery. This means a shorter battery life.

Open fit

Both BTE and RIC (or RITE) aids can be fit with a dome-shaped tip in the ear canal. This leaves the ear canal largely open. This style is commonly used for mild hearing loss and mild to moderate high-frequency hearing loss, for people who have typical or near-typical hearing in low frequencies. People with more severe hearing loss can't use the open-fit style because it doesn't offer enough volume and may cause feedback.

Because most of the ear canal is left open, individuals can use their remaining hearing for lower pitched sounds — which are able to pass directly to the eardrum — and the hearing aid selectively amplifies higher pitched sounds.

Advantages The ability of the casing to fit behind the ear, and the use of thin tubing or wire, makes the open-fit style attractive for those concerned about how a hearing aid looks. Leaving the ear canal open often makes the individual's own voice sound more natural.

Disadvantages This style is limited in how much volume it can produce before whistling or squealing (feedback) occurs.

Bone conduction devices

Sometimes, if the ear is poorly formed or there are medical problems with an ear, a conventional hearing aid won't work. A physical deformity or chronic drainage from the ear are examples.

In cases like these, devices that bypass the outer and middle ear and directly stimulate the inner ear can be used to overcome conductive hearing loss. These devices can also be used for single-sided deafness, when there's profound inner ear hearing loss in one ear and typical or near-typical hearing in the other ear.

A bone conduction device stimulates the inner ear with an external device that has a microphone and amplifier. This device changes sound to a vibration that's picked up by the inner ear. This device is sometimes called a bone-anchored hearing aid (BAHA) or a bone conduction system.

This type of device may be placed with or without surgery. A surgically placed device can be attached to a titanium post or implant behind the ear. Devices that aren't placed with surgery are attached to an elastic or metal headband or with an adhesive.

Advantages

Bone conduction devices can be used when conventional hearing aids that use air conduction aren't an option. Devices placed surgically or with adhesive are usually more comfortable than those attached to a headband.

Disadvantages

The external device that changes sound to a vibration that can be picked up by the inner ear can't be activated right after surgery. The wait time can vary from several weeks to several months. Feedback may be a bigger issue with a device that's attached to a headband. And repairs to the external device can be expensive if not covered by insurance.

Other implantable options

Other implantable hearing aids may be an option for people with moderate to severe hearing loss that's associated with damage to the inner ear.

These devices use a tiny electromagnet that's attached to the bones of the middle ear to amplify the sound wave going to the cochlea. These devices can be fully or partially implantable, meaning that the sound processor is either implanted under the skin or attached outside of the

head. This type of aid is not as common and is generally not covered by insurance. Ongoing research is still needed to determine its overall effectiveness.

OTHER CONSIDERATIONS

When choosing a hearing aid, you'll likely consider style, size and circuitry features. You may also need to decide if one hearing aid improves your hearing most, or if two hearing aids would help more. This process can get confusing because decisions regarding style, size and circuitry can be made somewhat independently of each other.

For example, you may have heard that digital hearing aids provide the best sound. What may not be clear is that *digital* refers to the electrical components, not to a particular style of hearing aid. All hearing aids now are digital.

Style and circuitry, along with size, are separate issues. Any circuitry can be placed in any style or size of hearing aid.

Here's more on considerations that may factor into a hearing aid choice.

Electronics

The circuitry of hearing aids refers to the electronic parts inside the casing. Hearing aid electronics are programmed to amplify some frequencies more than others depending on the results of your hearing test. Hearing aids are always monitoring the environment around you.

BONE CONDUCTION DEVICES

Here are examples of bone conduction devices, with details on how they work.

Bone-anchored hearing aid

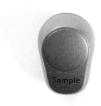
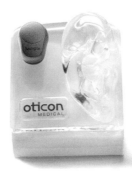

This type of device stimulates the inner ear with an external device that has a microphone and amplifier. This device changes sound to a vibration that's picked up by the inner ear. It may be placed with or without surgery.

Bone conduction device with adhesive adapter

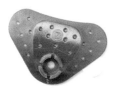
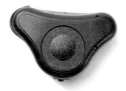
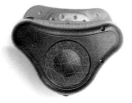

Bone conduction device adapter

Bone conduction device

Bone conduction device with adhesive adapter

With this newer type of device, a disposable adhesive adapter is placed onto the skin behind the ear. It connects to a bone conduction audio processor on your head. The adhesive allows the processor to stay in place without applying pressure to your head. The processor converts sound into vibrations that are transmitted via the adhesive adapter and relayed through the skin. Sound is then transmitted via bone conduction to the inner ear. This device doesn't require surgery and is used to treat conductive hearing loss and single-sided deafness in people of any age. The adhesive adapter lasts for 3 to 7 days.

Direct drive bone conduction implant

Placed fully under the skin, this implant works with an audio processor (pictured below) that sits on your head and can be hidden under your hair. Audio processors automatically change settings to make it easier to hear in difficult hearing environments, such as in traffic or in noisy restaurants. This type of device is intended for adults and children age 12 and older with mixed or conductive hearing loss, or single-sided deafness.

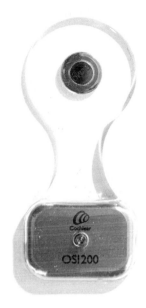

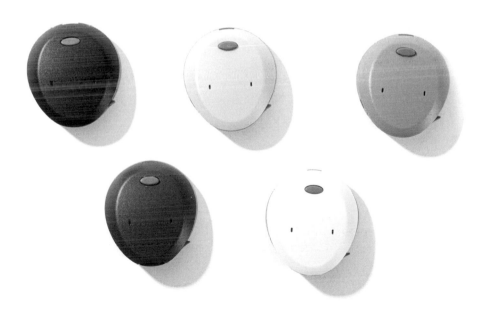

They are programmed to accommodate for different environments.

All of today's hearing aids are digital because they all have a small computer chip. Incoming sound is converted into a digital code. This digital code, in turn, is analyzed and adjusted based on your hearing loss and listening needs. The code is then converted back into sound waves and delivered to the ear canal. Computer chips make it so that sound is amplified more accurately. They also offer additional options in sound processing that make devices more comfortable to use in a variety of environments.

The computer chip lets the audiologist program the hearing aid to address your hearing loss and your personal preferences. For example, the chip allows the audiologist to adjust how much amplification is needed to hear at different frequencies or pitches. This depends on the type and severity of your hearing loss.

In addition, the computer chip can allow for several different settings for amplification. Some hearing aids make some of these changes automatically depending on changes in the environment. An audiologist can program one setting for use in quiet situations and another for use in loud, noisy situations, like restaurants or parties. With most hearing aids, you can choose a setting by pushing a small button on the outside of the hearing aid or, in some cases, with a cellphone or a remote control.

Often, special features can be activated for use in certain settings. For example,

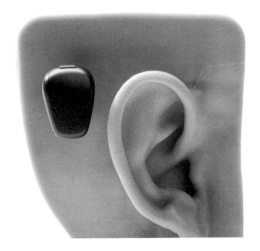

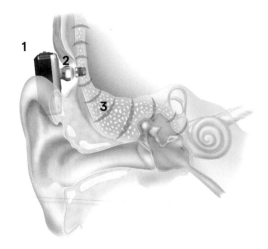

How a bone conduction device works: 1. The external processor receives sound waves and turns them into vibrations. 2. Vibrations from the sound processor are transferred to the titanium implant. 3. The implant uses direct bone conduction to transfer the sound vibrations to the functioning cochlea.

in noisy situations, you can activate directional microphones in the hearing aid that reduce the amount of noise that's picked up behind you (background noise). Your hearing aid will likely have special built-in noise-reduction circuitry. With most hearing aids, the computer chip's settings adjust automatically based on the amount of noise, where the noise is coming from and how loud sounds are.

Some new circuitry is available for people with severe or profound high-frequency hearing loss in cases when conventional hearing aids may not help. These hearing aid circuits shift or move high-frequency sounds to mid or low frequencies where the listener has better hearing and can "hear" the high-frequency sounds.

Some hearing aid circuitry allows devices worn in the right ear and the left ear to communicate with each other to make joint setting adjustments. Some options have wireless technology. This allows for better communication between hearing aids and cellphones or other electronic or Bluetooth devices.

The cost of digital hearing varies. Cost is determined mostly by how specific the amplification can get and how many special features and adjustments are included on the computer chip.

Typically, more-expensive hearing aids have more frequency bands or channels. The number of channels determines how well a hearing aid can be adjusted for the hearing loss and how parameters like noise reduction and feedback and other parameters are controlled.

For many people, less-expensive aids may offer enough features to suit their hearing loss and lifestyles. Other users may want all possible features and be willing to pay for them. Weigh the pros and cons against your needs and preferences.

Special options

Following are special options you may consider when choosing a hearing aid.

Directional microphones

A hearing aid may have many microphones that allow the hearing aid to switch between surround-sound and

WHAT IS FEEDBACK?

Feedback is the high-pitched whistle or squeal that happens when amplified sound is inadvertently picked up by the microphone and then re-amplified. This is similar to the loud noise you may hear over a speaker system when the volume is set too high. New technology is helping to reduce feedback problems in hearing aids.

directional modes. In fact, circuits in the most current hearing aids can make this switch automatically as the sound environment changes. All hearing aids except for CIC and some ITC styles can accommodate directional microphones.

Most directional microphones pick up sounds directly in front of you more than those coming from other directions. This helps the hearing aid take in less background noise and improve how well you hear someone you're face-to-face with.

Some new hearing aid circuits can be programmed to focus on sounds coming from other directions. For example, the aid can be right-focused so when you're driving, you can hear the person in the passenger seat next to you. Or it can be left-focused when you're riding in the passenger seat or rear-focused when you're driving with back-seat passengers.

Rechargeable batteries

Some hearing aids use rechargeable batteries. With one type, you can replace the battery yourself, either with another rechargeable battery or with a standard hearing aid battery. The other type uses a lithium-ion battery. It's sealed inside the hearing aid and has to be returned to the manufacturer for replacement.

The rechargeable hearing aid battery is available for behind-the-ear, receiver-in-canal, and in-the-ear and half-shell hearing aids. It usually comes with a charger that the hearing aid fits into. The charger will likely be either direct con-nection or inductive charging. Battery life per charge varies and depends on the amount of power the hearing aid has and how it's used. A lithium-ion battery typically holds a charge for approximately 16 to 20 hours and usually lasts about three years.

Telecoils

Many behind-the-ear aids, as well as some in-the-ear and ITC aids, have a built-in telecoil. A telecoil is a tiny metal rod encircled with a coil of copper wire. It picks up an electromagnetic signal from hearing-aid-compatible telephones and public address systems like those found in conference rooms, concert halls, museums and subway trains and converts that energy into sound. It allows you to hear someone clearly by telephone.

The telecoil can be manually activated with a switch, but many aids now have an internal switch that picks up the electromagnetic signal automatically when a hearing aid-compatible phone is held up to the hearing aid. When the telecoil is switched on, the microphone in the hearing aid can be turned off and only the telecoil signal is amplified. This prevents the feedback or squeal that often happens when a telephone is held close to a hearing aid with the microphone on.

Besides telephones, telecoils can be used with assistive listening systems (see Chapter 11). Current cellphones generally come with compatibility ratings for telecoils. The higher the number, the more compatible the cellphone is for hearing aids with a telecoil. The highest possible telecoil rating is T4.

Wireless connectivity

Many hearing aids can connect directly to other devices, typically through Bluetooth. Cellphones, tablets and smart televisions are examples.

Remote microphone

Some hearing aid companies offer a remote microphone that can be used with some hearing aids. The microphone is

HOW A TELECOIL WORKS

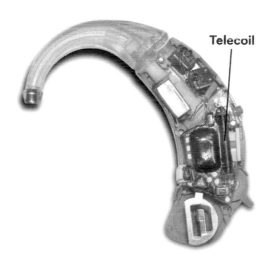

Telecoil

A telecoil picks up electromagnetic signals directly from the telephone receiver, allowing you to hear the caller's voice.

usually small and portable and can be passed to someone you're talking to.

Putting the microphone closer to the speaker's mouth places emphasis on the speaker's voice and significantly reduces environmental noise. This is helpful especially in noisy places or places where there is reverberation or echo.

Remote control

Some hearing aids can be operated with a remote control. This feature allows the user to turn the hearing aid on or off, and to adjust settings without touching the hearing aid or trying to find a small button or knob on it. Most companies now have a smartphone app that functions as a remote control.

Bluetooth interface

Some hearing aids have a type of streamer, used as a wireless interface between the hearing aid and Bluetooth devices like cellphones or other electronic devices. The streamer picks up the signal from the wireless device and sends it directly to the hearing aid. Streamers need to be kept close to the hearing aid and may come with a clip or cord to allow them to be worn around the neck. Some streamers can serve as a remote control.

Audio input

An input jack on the aid allows you to connect a wire directly to a television,

DEVICES YOU CAN USE WITH HEARING AIDS

Many hearing aids can be connected directly to other devices, typically through Bluetooth. Some hearing aids have a type of streamer, used as a wireless interface between the hearing aid and Bluetooth devices like cell-phones or other electronic devices. Here are several examples.

Television streaming device

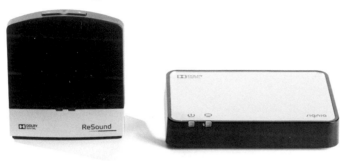

This device allows you to hear a television from a distance, at a comfortable volume, as long as you're in clear line of sight from it. It can be used for stereos and computers, as well.

Remote microphone

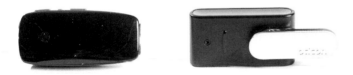

Remote microphones allow you to hear from a distance or in challenging environments, including lectures, houses of worship, business presentations and noisy restaurants. You simply place the microphone on a level surface like a table, and it picks up voices and allows you to hear them without having to wear a device around your neck. This is a device that you hand to someone you want to hear, like someone delivering a presentation or a friend you're having dinner with at a restaurant. This device can also transmit a call directly from your smartphone to your hearing aids.

Audio streaming device

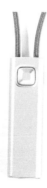

This hands-free device, which you wear around your neck, delivers sound to your hearing aid from someone you're talking to or any Bluetooth device.

Hearing aid remote control

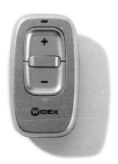

Some hearing aids can be operated with a remote control. This feature allows the user to turn the hearing aid on or off, and to adjust settings without touching the hearing aid or trying to find a small button or knob on it.

Hearing aid remote control and audio streaming device

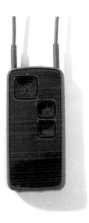

You can connect this device to a range of other devices. It allows you to hear a TV or to communicate through Bluetooth-enabled cellphones.

It can also serve as a remote control that enables you to adjust your hearing aid's volume and programming.

stereo, separate microphone or assistive listening device. This is an option on some behind-the-ear hearing aids, but not for styles worn inside the ear.

Ear-level FM systems

FM listening systems are especially helpful for overcoming the effects of background noise, reverberation and distance (see Chapter 11). Some behind-the-ear aids combine regular circuitry with an FM receiver in the same casing.

BUYING A HEARING AID

If you're planning to use hearing aids, it's best to talk with an audiologist or a hearing aid dispenser, also known as a hearing instrument specialist.

Audiologists need to earn a master's or doctoral degree in audiology (Au.D. or Ph.D.) to enter the practice. Licensing is required in all states in which they practice, and they may be certified by professional organizations like the American Speech-Language-Hearing Association or the American Academy of Audiology. The practices of many ear, nose and throat (ENT) specialists include audiologists on staff to provide testing and rehabilitation services and to dispense hearing aids.

Nonaudiologist hearing aid dispensers don't need a college degree. However, many complete coursework in the field. They're registered in the state they work in. In most states, hearing aid dispensers are licensed. This means they've passed state-administered examinations in the field. Dispensers are typically certified by the National Board for Certification in Hearing Instrument Sciences.

To find a reputable audiologist or hearing aid dispenser, ask your doctor. You can also get lists of qualified hearing professionals in your area by contacting hearing organizations like the American Academy of Audiology or the American Speech-

QUESTIONS TO ASK

When your audiologist or dispenser recommends a specific hearing aid, ask questions to understand why a certain hearing aid may be better for you than another. Here are several questions to ask:
- Why do you recommend this particular hearing aid?
- What is the benefit of this hearing aid over another?
- Why do you recommend this style of hearing aid for me?
- What is the return policy?
- What is the warranty?
- Is there a restocking fee if I return the hearing aids?

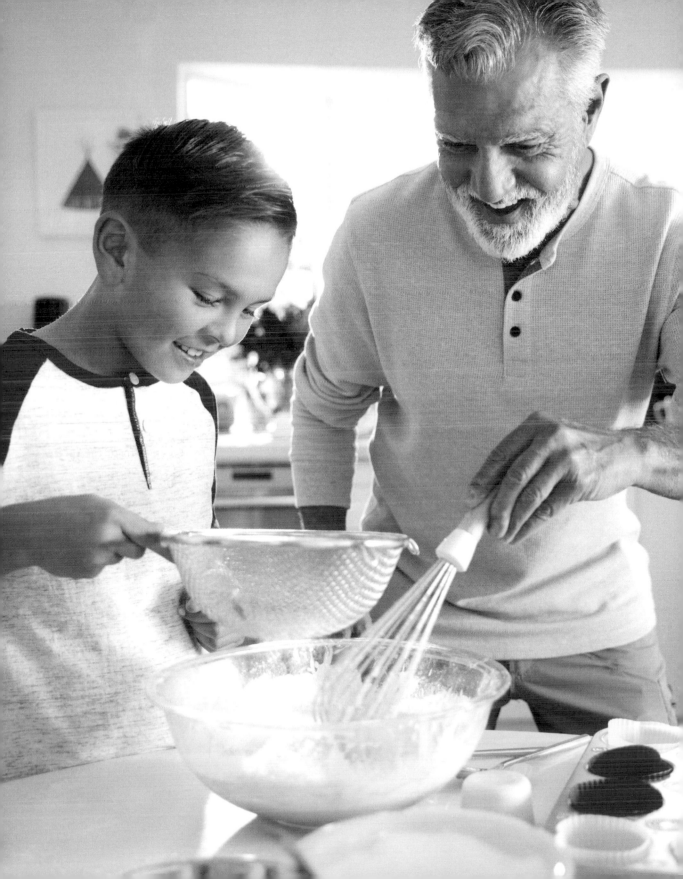

Language-Hearing Association (see the "Additional resources" chapter in this book for contact information). Several websites that sell hearing aids refer you to dispensers within their networks. Internet and mail-order hearing aid sales are illegal in several states.

Don't buy hearing aids by mail or via internet from makers who claim you don't need to see an audiologist or dispenser in person. Proper testing, fitting and adjustments are always essential parts of buying a hearing aid.

The buying process

Though the terms *hearing aid* and *aid* are used in the singular form in this chapter,

PURCHASING TIPS FOR HEARING AIDS

Keep the following suggestions in mind when selecting a hearing aid:
- Consider all the options available — more than one type of hearing aid might work for you. If your first selection doesn't work well for you, try a different one.
- Don't assume that the newest, most expensive model is the best for you. A less expensive aid might improve your hearing and be appropriate for you and your lifestyle.
- Be cautious of "free" consultations and dispensers who sell only one brand of hearing aid. Look for a dispenser who offers plenty of options from different manufacturers.
- Be alert to misleading claims. Be wary of ads that claim hearing aids can eliminate background noise or restore typical hearing. Most aids can help you, but no hearing aid can completely filter out one voice from other voices or restore your hearing.
- Ask what the cost of a hearing aid includes. A single fee may bundle the cost of the aid with the costs of follow-up visits, the warranty and one pack of batteries. Or, the charges may be unbundled, with professional fees separate from the charge for the hearing aid.
- Get the terms of the trial period and the warranty in writing. This typically includes the return policy, the amount that can be refunded, how long the warranty lasts (preferably at least one year), and specifically what is or isn't covered. The warranty also usually covers both parts and labor. Many warranties cover a one-time loss and damage replacement for a hearing aid.
- During the trial period, keep a detailed list of what you like or dislike about your hearing aid. Take the list with you when you return to the audiologist or dispenser.

you may choose to use a hearing aid in both ears. Often, people get the most hearing improvement with two aids.

To start the buying process, schedule a complete hearing evaluation by an audiologist. The exam helps determine if you need to see your doctor first before moving forward.

There are many reasons you may need to see your doctor before getting a hearing aid. They include:

- Confirming if something other than a hearing aid can improve your hearing
- Determining if a condition prevents you from being able to use a hearing aid
- Getting medical signoff for a hearing aid, which some health insurance plans require before paying for hearing aids

Talk about your needs and expectations with your audiologist or hearing aid dispenser. Discuss which situations are the most difficult. The goal is to match lifestyle and communication needs as closely as possible.

After studying the evaluation of your hearing loss and considering lifestyle needs, the audiologist or dispenser usually offers several options and recommendations. Make sure you understand why a specific type of hearing aid has been recommended. Find questions to ask on page 154.

Before making a final decision, get to know all the features, as well as the cost, the terms of the trial period and the return policy. Hearing aids usually come with a trial period and a return policy. A trial period gives you time to adjust to using the device and decide whether it helps your hearing enough to keep it. After you've made a selection, the audiologist or dispenser fits the hearing aid. For some styles, an impression of the ear will be made with a puttylike material. This helps the manufacturer make a custom ear mold or hearing aid that is comfortable and fits properly in the ear.

After 1 to 3 weeks, you'll return to the audiologist or dispenser's office to

BUYING HEARING AIDS OVER THE COUNTER

Over-the-counter (OTC) hearing aids are a new category of hearing aids that you may soon have the option to buy. A law was recently passed that allows the Food and Drug Administration to create this new category of hearing aids so that more adults have access to hearing aid devices.

Over-the-counter hearing aids are meant for adults who believe they have mild to moderate hearing loss. These devices are not meant for children or anyone with more-severe degrees of hearing loss. The Food and Drug Administration is establishing regulations for manufacturers to follow.

resume the fitting process. This time, you'll wear the hearing aid. The audiologist typically programs or adjusts the aid to ensure it offers the most assistance. The best way to verify that the hearing aid is adjusted properly is by measuring how it amplifies sound. This is done by playing speech or other sounds from a speaker and measuring what comes out of the hearing aid with several microphones and a tube that sits in the ear canal. This measurement is called a real-ear measure because it is actually measuring what the hearing aid does to sound in the ear.

Once the hearing aid is fit and programmed, the audiologist or dispenser

GRETA'S STORY: KEEP A POSITIVE ATTITUDE

When Greta was 8 years old, she failed a hearing screening at school. Although her hearing loss was mild at the time, she was wearing hearing aids in both ears by age 13.

Now, as an adult, Greta has years of experience under her belt with bilateral sensorineural hearing loss. She also has experience with hearing loss in another way — as a Mayo Clinic audiologist. Greta diagnoses and helps people cope with hearing loss every day.

While you may feel that the term *hearing loss* means that you are missing something that everyone else has, Greta says it doesn't have to be seen as a bad thing. "Some people approach it as, 'There's something wrong or different with me,' or, 'I don't want anyone to see that I'm wearing a hearing aid.' Hearing loss only means that you might need a different set of circumstances in order to achieve the same performance as someone else," Greta says. And, she adds, hearing loss is much more common than people realize.

With this in mind, your attitude can make all the difference. However, if you see hearing aids in the same way you see glasses, it's likely that you'll be frustrated.

"Hearing aids are *aids*," Greta says. "They help and they can provide a lot of benefit, but underneath it, there's still a damaged auditory system. You're sometimes going to have some struggles. You might have times when you need to modify your environment or use assistive listening devices to hear differently. Having a positive attitude and a set of communication strategies to use will help you maximize your hearing abilities."

will usually teach you how to use and maintain it. You'll likely be shown how to insert and remove the device, check the battery, adjust the controls, and keep it clean and operational.

You'll likely sign a purchase agreement. Be sure to read the agreement carefully and ask any questions before signing it.

About the trial period

A trial period gives you time to adjust to the hearing aid. You'll probably schedule a return visit or two to the office within a few weeks. If you have ear pain or discomfort or you can't use the hearing aid, call your audiologist's or dispenser's office to ask if you should come in sooner.

One of your biggest assets in your hearing loss journey will be your audiologist, Greta says. She experienced this firsthand; her first audiologist wasn't a good fit and didn't provide the encouragement she needed. Finding a new audiologist made all the difference.

"My new audiologist explained everything as we went through the process and made me feel like I was an integral part of the decision-making. He made me feel valued and recognized me as a part of the solution," Greta says.

Now, as an audiologist herself, Greta strives to give the same encouragement and support — and even a little bit of excitement — to her patients.

"A lot of times when I'm bringing patients back, I say, 'So are you excited to get your new hearing aids today?' I make it as fun as possible," Greta says.

While Greta understands that people may not jump for joy over getting hearing aids, she says there truly is reason to be excited. "I see so many people when they come back for their first follow-up appointment, and they're like, 'Gosh, why didn't I do this sooner?'"

The key, Greta says, is to find an audiologist you can truly partner with.

"You need to see your audiologist as your cheerleader, as your coach and as your teammate," Greta says. "You need to help them know what's most important to you. How do you want to hear better? Where are you struggling? What's important to you? Having that relationship and that safe environment to really be able to share that — that is so, so key."

Before your appointment, write down any questions or concerns you have. Take them to your appointment.

If during the trial period you can't adjust to the aid or you decide that it doesn't help you hear better, let your audiologist or dispenser know. The purchase agreement generally spells out how to return a hearing aid and what charges are associated with the trial period. These terms vary from state to state.

Costs

The cost of a hearing aid varies considerably. Most digital aids range from $1,500 to more than $3,000 apiece. With two aids, the costs about double.

Although this may sound expensive, only you can say whether hearing aids are worth the cost — in other words, if they'll help you hear better and improve your quality of life, making them worth the investment.

Medicare and many private insurance policies don't cover the cost of a hearing aid. However, in recent years, more employer- and union-sponsored policies have started providing limited coverage or reimbursement.

Veterans may be eligible for free hearing aids and services, as well as batteries and other accessories, through the Veterans Affairs. Some fraternal and charitable organizations provide financial assistance for hearing aids for people who meet financial eligibility requirements.

WEARING A HEARING AID

You'll likely notice immediate improvement in the first days of wearing a hearing aid, but more benefits come after you've gotten used to the device.

Getting used to a hearing aid takes patience and practice. The brain requires time to readjust to sounds that you may not have heard for a while. Some sounds may seem different when they're amplified by the device.

To get the most benefit from a hearing aid, it's important to understand how it works, learn to insert it properly and use it regularly. A positive attitude also helps.

Schedule follow-up appointments. After a week or two, you may want to have it adjusted or fine-tuned based on everyday experiences or for better comfort and control. An audiologist or hearing aid dispenser helps you achieve the best fit and greatest benefit.

The audiologist or hearing aid dispenser usually continues to help you with operating and maintaining the aid. Practice using your hearing aid when you're with your audiologist or hearing aid dispenser. If you use two aids, practice inserting and removing both aids. The hearing aids and ear molds are identified using red and blue. Red is always for the right ear and blue is always for the left ear. Practice adjusting the controls, cleaning the aid and changing the batteries. The more you practice using and taking care of your hearing aids, the easier it will likely become.

Adjustment

When you first use a hearing aid, some sounds may not seem natural. With the use of an aid, you'll likely hear more — and louder — sounds.

Many first-time hearing aid users say that people's voices, including their own, sound strange. The voices you hear are picked up by a microphone and amplified. Hearing aids are programmed to amplify certain pitches more than others depending on your degree of hearing loss — so you may be hearing sounds that you haven't heard for some time. However, the more you wear the aid, the sooner sounds will seem natural to you.

As your hearing has decreased over the years, you've probably gotten used to a quieter life. Many common environmental sounds, like appliance motors, clocks, dripping faucets, a car's running motor, footsteps, even your own chewing or breathing, were soft or too soft to hear when you weren't using a hearing aid.

During the first days of wearing a hearing aid, you'll likely start noticing these sounds again. Because you haven't heard them for a while, your brain may be more aware of them. The change may be annoying at first. But after several weeks and months, the brain will likely shift these sounds to the background where they belong, and you'll notice them less.

TIPS FOR FRIENDS AND FAMILY

Communication is a two-way street. Those who don't have hearing loss can communicate well with those who do by using these tips.

- Get the person's attention before talking.
- Face the person.
- Stay within a few feet of the person.
- Speak as loudly as you usually do or a little louder. Don't shout.
- Speak just a little more slowly than usual.
- Limit background noise. Turn off the TV or radio.
- Be sure you have good lighting, so you can see each other's faces.
- Talk one-on-one, rather than in a group setting.
- Repeat what you said. Then say it again in a little different way. Hearing in a different way can help a person's understanding.
- Pause and ask if you're being heard.
- Review key points at the end of the conversation.
- Let the listener know when you're going to change the topic.
- Write out things that are hard to understand.
- Include your listener. Ask for opinions and comments. Taking an active part in conversation improves communication.

Most audiologists recommend using a new hearing aid during most of your waking hours. If you're having a problem adjusting to the aid, consider using it only for a few hours a day at home, where you can control the noise level. Practice talking with one or two people in a quiet place. Then increase the amount of time you use the aid each day little by little.

As your comfort level builds, expose yourself to different listening situations until you're able to use your aid all day in any environment. It may take some time — maybe months — to get used to new sounds and get the most out of the hearing aid.

Discuss any problems with your audiologist or hearing aid dispenser. You may be directed to a group orientation session for new hearing aid users. This session provides information about hearing loss and hearing aid use.

You may also contact an organization like the Hearing Loss Association of America (find contact information in the "Additional resources" section of this book).

Tips for better communication

Hearing aids are meant to improve communication, not to give you new ears or the hearing of a typical 20-year-old. You'll inevitably find times in which hearing aids don't give you all of the benefits you'd like.

In these situations, you may need to rely on additional methods to improve communication. When needed, consider adding these strategies:

Don't talk to people from a different room

Distance and barriers like walls reduce the amount of sound that reaches you.

Talk face-to-face

When you're talking to someone, make sure you can see his or her face and lips. Converse on a one-to-one basis or in small groups rather than large groups.

Control background noise

Talk in locations with the least background noise. Steer clear of noisy restaurants, or go during off-peak times to avoid a crowd. You may also ask for a booth in a quiet corner with good lighting. In meeting rooms and lecture halls, sit in the front row. At home, turn off the television or stereo while talking on the phone or in person.

Ask others to help

People are usually glad to accommodate you if they understand your needs. Let others know how to help you and what listening strategies work for you.

Start by telling people that the circumstances are making it tough for you to hear. Ask them to talk directly to you face-to-face and to speak clearly and slowly, but remind them it's not necessary to shout.

Learn about other assistive tools, including devices and listening systems

Resources like a telephone amplifier, FM system, Bluetooth technology, induction loop or closed captioning service may help in difficult listening environments. Learn about them in Chapter 11.

Common problems

As with any complex piece of equipment, things can go wrong with a hearing aid.

Most problems are minor and easy to correct.

It's always important to inform your audiologist or hearing aid dispenser of any problem. Before calling, however, see if the problem is something that you can easily fix:

- Is the hearing aid turned on?
- Are all switches or controls in the correct position?
- Is the battery fresh and inserted properly?
- Is the sound outlet plugged with earwax or debris?
- Is the microphone opening plugged?
- If you have a remote control for the aid, is it functioning?

BATTERY BASICS

- Use only the size and type of battery recommended by your audiologist or hearing aid dispenser.
- Most hearing aid batteries are zinc-air. They're activated when an adhesive tab is removed and air gets into the battery. Never remove the tab until you're ready to insert the battery into your hearing aid.
- Zinc-air batteries have an excellent shelf life, so you can keep several packages on hand.
- Store your batteries at room temperature, not in a refrigerator.
- Battery life depends on the style and circuitry of the hearing aid, the size of battery and how many hours a day the aid is used. Most hearing aid batteries last from 5 to 7 days, although small batteries last only about 2 to 4 days. At your initial fitting, talk about creating a battery replacement schedule.
- You can buy batteries from your audiologist or hearing aid dispenser, in drugstores, grocery stores and electronics supply stores via internet.
- Keep batteries out of reach of children and pets, and dispose of them properly. Ask your audiologist about any battery-recycling rules and regulations.

Here are tips for some of the most common problems with hearing aids.

Earwax

The most common cause of hearing aid failure is earwax. People who don't wear hearing aids can get earwax buildup, but it gradually loosens, moves to the edge of the ear canal and falls out.

If you wear a hearing aid, placing the aid or ear mold in your ear can stimulate earwax production. A hearing aid or ear mold can compress the earwax and cause it to stay in the canal. Earwax can plug the piece that sits in the ear canal and block sound.

The best way to prevent earwax buildup is to visit a doctor or audiologist regularly to have the earwax removed. It's a simple procedure. Don't try to remove the earwax by using cotton swabs. This may pack the earwax deeper into the ear canal and damage the eardrum. Ask your audiologist or hearing aid dispenser about how to keep earwax from getting inside your hearing aids, such as an earwax guard. He or she can show you the best way to clean earwax from the aid. Every day, inspect the end of the hearing aid where the sound comes out and look for earwax blockage.

Dead or defective batteries

The second most common cause of hearing aid failure is a weak or dead battery. Weak output, distortion, in-creased feedback, and other strange or unusual sounds, such as crackling static or fluttering are common signs that a battery may be failing.

If you notice any of these signs, try inserting a new battery or charging the battery or hearing aid. When you replace the battery, make sure that the battery is placed correctly with the plus sign facing in the right direction. Most hearing aids give you a warning tone that your battery needs to be replaced or recharged.

Feedback

Whistling and squealing are usually the result of a poorly fit hearing aid, an improperly inserted device or an ear that's plugged with earwax. The more powerful a hearing aid is, the more critical the fit is for receiving and amplifying sound.

When you experience feedback, always check for the following:
- Make sure the aid is inserted properly in your ear.
- Make sure the volume control isn't set too high.
- Have your audiologist or doctor check your ear for earwax buildup.

Ear discomfort

The ear mold of a behind-the-ear aid or the shell of custom hearing aids usually fits snugly in the ear but isn't uncomfortable. At first the ear mold or hearing aid may feel slightly uncomfortable, but it shouldn't cause soreness, redness or irritation. Discomfort may also result from poor fit or from an aid that's positioned incorrectly in the ear canal. Difficulties with placement are fairly common among new hearing aid users.

If you experience constant discomfort from wearing an aid, stop using it and talk to your audiologist or dispenser about the problem. The ear mold or hearing aid may need to be modified or remade.

Moisture

Moisture often collects in the tubing between the ear mold and the behind-the-ear casing. As warm air from the inside of the ear travels into the cooler tubing, water vapor condenses and collects in the tubing.

This usually isn't a problem unless the tubing becomes plugged. Moisture, like sweat on the skin behind the ear, also can affect a behind-the-ear aid. It can affect in-the-ear hearing aids, too. Storing aids in a dehumidifier pack may help. Electronic drying devices also are available.

Maintenance

Proper care is key to keeping a hearing aid in good working order. Here are a few suggestions.

Keep the hearing aid clean and dry

Wipe your hearing aid with a tissue or soft cloth every time you take it out of your ear. Gently scrub it with a soft brush every morning before inserting it. This is when earwax is dry and crumbles and falls out more easily.

Keep the hearing aid charged

For hearing aids with rechargeable batteries, put the hearing aid in the charger nightly. The hearing aid doesn't need to be turned off when it's in the charger.

Check the small holes at the tip of the hearing aid or custom ear mold

Carefully clean out any earwax with a small brush, a wire looped around the end of a piece of plastic (a wax loop) or a pick. Most custom hearing aids that fit in the ear have a built-in earwax guard. RIC and RITE hearing aid receivers that fit in the ear canal have them, too. Earwax guards can be replaced at home or in the dispenser's office.

Keep the hearing aid in a safe, dry, dust-free space

You may want to buy a dehumidifying container to store it in at night. Ask your dispenser to recommend a container.

Have the hearing aid cleaned and serviced regularly

Never try to repair a hearing aid yourself. You may damage the aid and void the

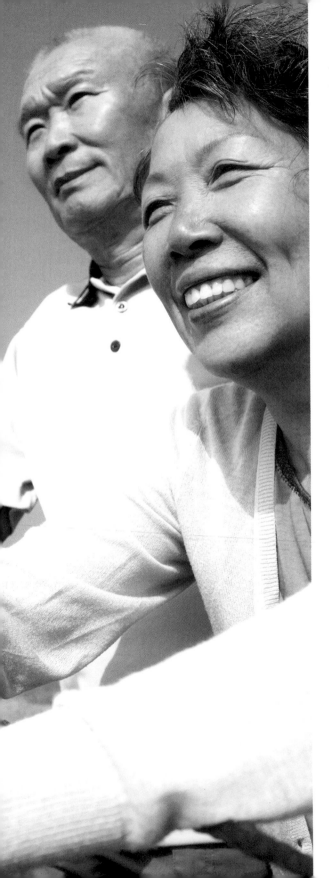

warranty. If the hearing aid breaks or isn't working, contact your audiologist or hearing aid dispenser. It's a good idea to have hearing aids checked out once a year to make sure they're working well.

Don't drop the hearing aid

Develop a habit of inserting and removing the aid over a soft surface, like a bed or sofa, or over a hand towel on a table. Never leave the aid where it could be knocked to the floor.

Don't wear your aid while bathing, showering or swimming

Also keep it away from steamy kitchens or bathrooms where someone has just taken a shower. Don't spray it with hair spray.

Don't expose the hearing aid to intense heat

Don't leave the aid on the top of a warm or hot surface, and don't leave it in the car when it's parked in the sun. Don't use the oven or microwave to dry out your hearing aid.

PHOTO QUIZ: HOW DID YOU SCORE?

As you looked through the photos in this chapter, how many people do you think were wearing hearing aids? If you said all of them, you are correct!

For hearing aids that use regular hearing aid batteries, keep the battery door open when the hearing aid isn't in use

This ensures that the hearing aid is turned off. It also lets dry air in and moisture out and saves battery life.

Keep batteries away from children and pets

Always keep the hearing aid and the batteries away from small children and pets. They can choke on an aid or swallow a battery. Batteries can also damage the body, burning holes in parts of the digestive system. Call the **National Battery Ingestion Hotline** at **1-800-498-8666** if you think a battery has been swallowed.

Make it routine

Get into a habit of putting the hearing aid in the same place every time you take it off. This will help make it less likely that you'll misplace or lose it.

BENEFITS BEYOND BETTER HEARING

Hearing aids can improve hearing, but they don't stop there. Some studies suggest that they also help with the depression, distress and anxiety that often accompanies hearing loss.

Likewise, people with hearing loss who wear hearing aids are less lonely and more socially active than those who don't.

As you consider looking into hearing aids or if you're adjusting to life with them, keep these benefits in mind. They may provide the encouragement you need as you choose a hearing aid and gradually make it a part of your life.

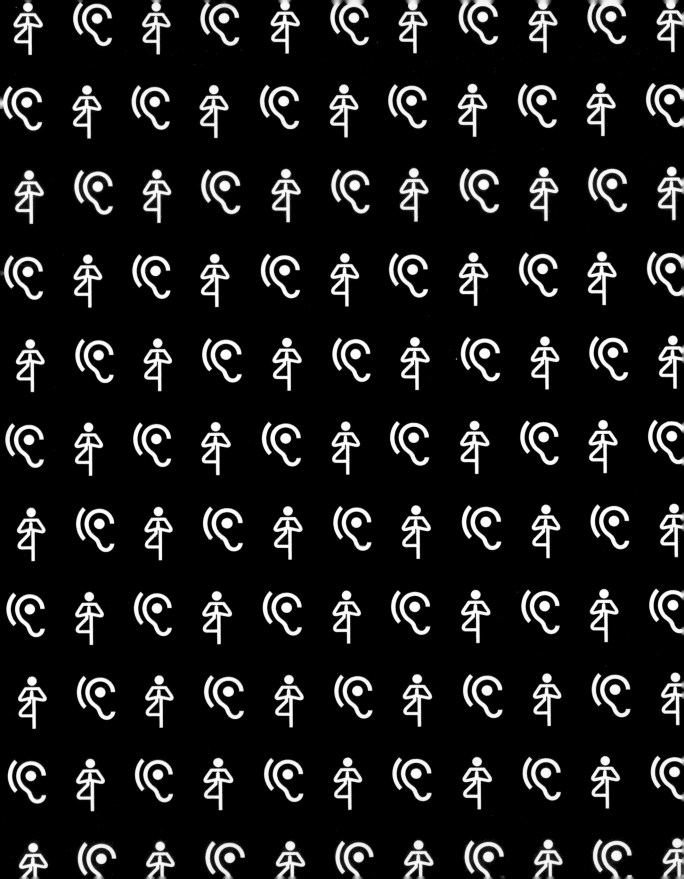

Cochlear implants

10

When Judith turned 50, she started to lose her hearing. After a visit to an audiologist, Judith started wearing hearing aids. They helped at first, but over time, Judith's hearing got worse, even with the aids.

That's when her audiologist suggested a cochlear implant.

Initially, Judith was apprehensive about risking what natural hearing she still had. "I was worried that if the cochlear implant didn't work, I would lose all the hearing in my left ear," Judith said.

Over the next few years, Judith's hearing continued to worsen. "I was missing out on life," she said. After much thought and many conversations with her health care team, Judith decided to move forward

with cochlear implant surgery. Judith's surgery went well, and one month afterward, the hearing in her left ear was up to 70%.

"I'm myself again," Judith said. "And it's just so wonderful."

Sensorineural hearing loss results from damage to the inner ear and to the auditory nerve that carries signals to the brain. The damage is usually permanent, and the hearing loss is irreversible.

Currently, the most effective treatment for adults and children with moderate to profound sensorineural hearing loss and poor understanding of speech is a cochlear implant. A cochlear implant is an electronic device that generates a sense of sound by stimulating the hearing nerve. This can help people who would gain little to no benefit from the amplified sound of hearing aids.

A cochlear implant is like an artificial inner ear, taking over the job of the cochlea. A healthy cochlea converts sound waves into electrical signals. It then sends those signals along the auditory nerve. If the cochlea is damaged, an implant can be surgically placed in the inner ear that directly stimulates the auditory nerve. An external device then picks up the sound and transmits it to the internal device.

Research on cochlear implants began in the 1950s as scientists looked to help people with sensorineural hearing loss. They began experimenting with ways to compensate for the damaged hair cells in the inner ear. The first devices were approved for adults in 1985 and for children in 1990.

Cochlear implant technology has improved tremendously since its introduction more than three decades ago, and new developments are on the horizon. Hundreds of thousands of adults and children around the world have benefitted from the procedure and are using the implants in their daily lives.

Although a cochlear implant doesn't restore lost hearing, it can dramatically improve your ability to hear and to understand speech. Benefits vary from person to person, but some users find that it allows them to perform many tasks that previously were difficult, like talking on the phone or listening in a classroom.

Hearing with a cochlear implant is different from typical hearing, and it takes the brain time to make sense of the information it's receiving. With consistent use, understanding will likely improve. After a few months or so of using the implant, the recipient usually finds that the sound of other voices begins to seem natural. For children with hearing loss since birth or a very young age, cochlear implants provide enough hearing input to develop speech and language.

Many people with cochlear implants experience a boost in their quality of life. The new sense of sound helps reduce feelings of isolation and helps them participate in social situations. They're able to enjoy pleasurable sounds such as the laughter of babies and — sometimes with time — the harmonies of song. They feel safer because they can hear fire alarms, warning sirens and traffic noise. They can better perform their jobs by being able to hear the ring of a telephone or the beep of a timer and to participate more one-on-one or in group meetings.

COCHLEAR IMPLANTS VS. HEARING AIDS

A cochlear implant is very different from a hearing aid. Hearing aids amplify sound waves, making them stronger when they're delivered to the ear. This amplification helps make more sounds detectable, louder and understandable.

Instead of making sounds louder, a cochlear implant bypasses the parts of the inner ear that are damaged or aren't working and stimulates the auditory nerve directly. The implant gathers acoustic information from the environment around you and converts it into a form that your brain can understand.

Usually, the sensory hair cells in the inner ear convert sound vibrations arriving from the middle ear into nerve impulses. These impulses are relayed to the brain. The brain interprets the impulses and gives them meaning as sounds.

In order for a person to hear sounds correctly, thousands of tiny hair cells must be functioning in the inner ear to fully detect the vibrations. A person with typical hearing will usually have about 16,000 healthy, delicate hair cells in each ear.

In most people with sensorineural hearing loss, some hair cells are damaged and don't function properly. They're unable to stimulate the auditory nerve effectively. Although many nerve fibers are intact and able to transmit electrical impulses, these fibers are unresponsive because of the hair cell damage.

People with mild or moderate hearing loss still typically have enough healthy hair cells to hear. Undamaged hair cells can still process sounds that are amplified by a hearing aid and convert them into electrical impulses that can be sent to the brain, like in a typical-hearing ear.

But if you have moderate to profound sensorineural hearing loss, your hair cells may be too damaged for your hearing system to process sound, no matter how much hearing aids amplify it.

Cochlear implants help resolve this because they're able to stimulate the intact nerve fibers directly. This allows you to communicate auditory information to your brain and perceive sounds.

HOW COCHLEAR IMPLANTS WORK

The Food and Drug Administration (FDA) has approved several cochlear implant systems and is testing others. All of them work by converting sounds into electronic impulses that are transmitted to your brain.

Cochlear implants have internal and external components. A microphone, speech processor, transmitter and connecting cords make up the external parts. The internal components are a receiver-stimulator and electrodes. Here's how the parts of a cochlear implant work together:

- A microphone is located in a headpiece or casing that's typically hooked over the ear, similar to a behind-the-ear hearing aid. The microphone picks up sounds from the environment.
- A sound processor takes the sounds picked up by the microphone and converts them into electronic impulses. Processors are often worn behind the ear, like a hearing aid. They can also be clipped to a shirt, armband or hat. A newer style incorporates the microphone, processor and transmitter into a single casing worn on the head over the internal receiver-stimulator.

- Impulses from the sound processor are sent to a transmitter, sometimes called a transmitting coil. A magnet holds the transmitter in place behind the ear, directly over a receiver-stimulator that's implanted beneath the scalp.
- The receiver-stimulator receives the impulses as radiofrequency waves from the transmitter. It relays the impulses as electronic signals through electrodes to the inner ear. The electrodes have been threaded directly into the cochlea on a bundle of tiny insulated wires.
- The electrodes stimulate the intact nerve fibers in the cochlea. This triggers the creation of electrical impulses. The impulses travel along the auditory nerve to the brain. Once the impulses reach the brain, the sound is interpreted and you understand what you've heard.

While this process may seem complicated, it takes only a fraction of a second from start to finish.

WHO SHOULD USE A COCHLEAR IMPLANT?

Research on cochlear implants is ongoing. Although cochlear implants work well for many people, some people don't do as well with them and have trouble with speech recognition, even after several years of use and rehabilitation.

Researchers are studying this issue to find out why cochlear implants don't always work well and how these devices can be improved. Researchers are also interested in pinpointing factors that make cochlear implants work well for some and not for others — before a person gets an implant.

Cochlear implants aren't alternatives to hearing aids. These devices are best for people when hearing aids provide little or no benefit.

Candidates for cochlear implants typically have moderate to profound sensorineural hearing loss in both ears or have great difficulty understanding speech. However, the criteria for implantation have changed significantly over the years.

Traditionally, people best suited for cochlear implants had been those with severe to profound hearing loss in both ears (bilateral) caused by damage to the inner ear (sensorineural). But advances in cochlear implant technology now make these devices suitable for people who have high-frequency hearing loss but can still hear low-frequency sounds. There are even hybrid devices that combine the technology of a cochlear implant and that a hearing aid in the same unit.

The earliest age for implantation in children can vary. Although cochlear implants are approved by the FDA for use in children at 9 to 12 months of age, some large centers have implanted them in children at 6 months.

In general, the younger a child is at the time of implantation, the less delay there will be in speech and language development — so long as appropriate therapy and education are provided after the procedure. Research shows that children

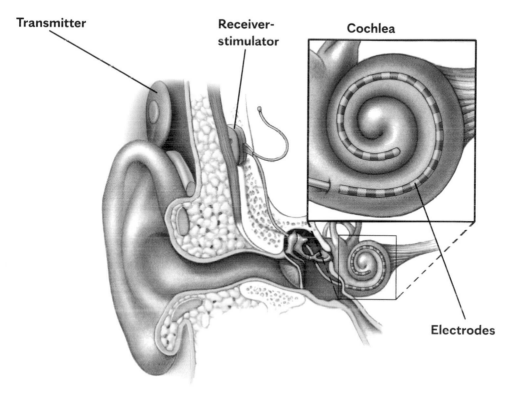

Transmitter

Receiver-
stimulator

Cochlea

Electrodes

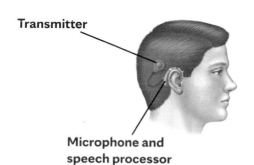

Transmitter

Microphone and
speech processor

Cochlear implants use an external microphone and speech processor that you generally wear behind or near your ear. A
transmitter sends radiofrequency signals
to a surgically implanted electronic chip,
the receiver-stimulator, that stimulates the
auditory nerve with electrodes that have
been threaded into the cochlea.

A   B   C

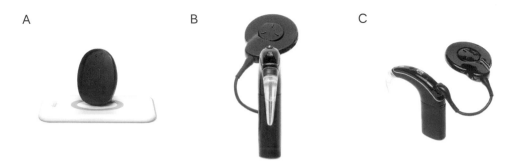

Above are two different external component styles for cochlear implants. Processors are most often worn behind the ear, similar to a hearing aid (B, C). These processors can also be worn using a clip pinned to a shirt, armband or hat.

A newer style of processor incorporates the microphone, processor and transmitter into a single casing that's worn on the head over the internal receiver-stimulator (A).

Below is a typical receiver-stimulator used with the different types of cochlear implants. The receiver-stimulator receives impulses as radiofrequency waves from the transmitter. It relays the impulses as electronic signals through electrodes to the inner ear.

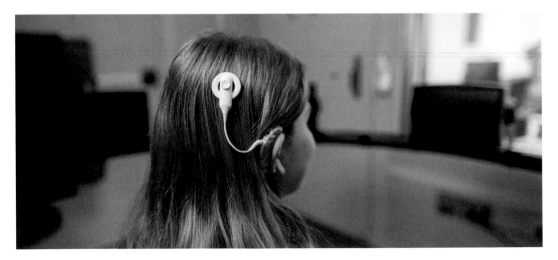

who get cochlear implants before age 2 typically have the most success hearing with the device.

There's no upper age limit for adults; even people in their 90s get cochlear implants. Studies indicate that people older than age 65 can experience excellent outcomes, with significant benefits for both communication and awareness of the environment.

Cochlear implants require careful consideration. In addition to having hearing loss, candidates must:
• Have realistic expectations — a clear understanding of the benefits and limitations of the implant

COCHLEAR IMPLANTS AND THE DEAF COMMUNITY

The Deaf community in the United States is a vibrant culture that includes a shared language (American Sign Language) and lifestyle and social customs, as well as educational, economic, artistic and recreational institutions and organizations. Members of the Deaf community don't view hearing loss as a disability that should be cured but as a cultural identity that's an important part of who they are. Because of this, many in the Deaf community do not support the use of cochlear implants, especially for children.

However, not all individuals who are deaf participate in Deaf culture. In fact, most children with profound hearing loss are born to parents with typical hearing. This has been a contentious issue for parents who were born deaf because children usually receive implants at such a young age. Some parents have received negative reactions for choosing a cochlear implant for their child rather than integrating into Deaf culture.

Both perspectives are valid, and many people recognize the value of being fluent in both hearing and Deaf cultures. Deaf and hearing-impaired people can continue to remain part of Deaf culture, but a cochlear implant allows them to have greater participation in the hearing community. Some Deaf individuals have found that a cochlear implant can help with environmental awareness, like the ability to hear alarms or a child crying.

If you, your child or a family member has profound hearing loss, you may find it helpful to talk to people with different viewpoints. Ask questions of those who use cochlear implants, those who use sign language and spoken language, and those who oppose cochlear implants. These discussions can help you better understand the different perspectives and choose the best option.

- Be willing to commit to the pre-implant evaluations and post-surgical follow-up services
- Be motivated for the change, with the support of family and friends

The decision to receive an implant should be made only after discussing it with a cochlear implant audiologist and an experienced cochlear implant surgeon. These are the experts most equipped to help you make this decision.

Contributing factors

Although there's no way to predict how well a cochlear implant will work, many factors can contribute to success.

Duration of hearing loss

People who've had moderate to profound hearing loss for a relatively short period of time usually adapt to an implant more readily. Those who've had profound hearing loss since birth or since they were very young typically have a harder time adjusting. In general, the shorter the duration of hearing loss, the better the outcome. People with some residual hearing or progressive (rather than sudden) hearing loss tend to have more success with cochlear implants.

Auditory nerve fibers

People with a greater number of functioning nerve fibers in the cochlea may benefit more from a cochlear implant. No test can determine an exact number or location of functioning fibers, but imaging tests such as magnetic resonance imaging (MRI) and computerized tomography (CT) may provide valuable clues to the cochlear implant surgeon.

Sometimes, an electrical stimulation test can check the auditory nerve to see if it will respond to small electrical signals.

Motivation

Much of the success of a cochlear implant depends on motivation and support. This commitment requires you to use the implant full time, maintain it, keep follow-up appointments and take advantage of rehabilitation strategies.

Counseling is an important part of the process. A cochlear implant is a tool, not a miracle cure. It will not restore hearing, but will give you the means to hear. Counseling can provide you with realistic expectations of the procedure.

Support

People who have a strong support network tend to adjust better to life with a cochlear implant than those who don't.

Benefits

According to reports from new users, sounds heard with a cochlear implant can range from being "tinny" and "computer-like" to being almost like typical sounds.

Generally, implant recipients notice the most improvement in the first year of using the device. But improvements can continue for many years after.

Adult cochlear implant users generally can communicate more effectively and with less effort. Most recipients who are profoundly deaf are able to detect soft sounds, including quiet speech, and recognize many everyday noises. For some people, the benefits are even greater. Detecting voices from another room, talking on the phone and enjoying music are all possible.

For many children, a cochlear implant has an impact on their potential to develop spoken language. Many can receive most of their education without the use of sign language or other methods of speech representation.

In general, adults with cochlear implants are significantly better able to understand speech. The level of improvement can

COSTS AND BENEFITS

The cost of getting a cochlear implant — including pre-implant evaluation, surgery and hospital fees; medical personnel fees; implant hardware; and post-surgical fittings and training — can run in the tens of thousands of dollars.

But unlike hearing aids, cochlear implants are often covered by private insurance plans as well as Medicare and Medicaid programs. In some states, coverage is provided by children's special services, Tricare or state vocational rehabilitation agencies. Many people receive support from community or charitable organizations that hold special fundraisers, like the Lions Club, Kiwanis, Sertoma and Jaycees.

Implant centers will likely have an insurance or reimbursement specialist who can help you determine the coverage provided by your health plan and assist you with obtaining pre-authorization for coverage. It's important that you start the process early and allow your insurance company sufficient time to review your information before proceeding.

Many researchers who have studied the cost-effectiveness of cochlear implants find that these devices greatly improve quality of life for those with significant hearing loss. They suggest considering cochlear implants not just in terms of what they cost but also in terms of how well the device can help you communicate and enhance your overall well-being. Cochlear implants may also help you rely less on special resources and support services.

vary; experts are still learning why people differ in terms of how much speech they understand. Overall it's expected that you'll have reasonable speech understanding within a few months after surgery. When the speech occurs in a personal conversation or within a familiar context, the level of understanding is even better — especially if the conversation is direct and face to face.

THE IMPLANT PROCEDURE

A thorough evaluation of how you hear with and without well-fit hearing aids is the first step. This will guide many decisions you and your doctor make. After the device has been implanted and activated, a series of follow-up sessions are necessary for fine-tuning of the device and speech perception testing.

COCHLEAR IMPLANTS AND DEAFNESS IN ONE EAR

For many years, it was thought that people with single-sided deafness couldn't benefit from cochlear implants. Single-sided deafness is severe or profound hearing loss in one ear and typical hearing in the other. Experts had hypothesized that the brain would have difficulties processing both typical hearing and hearing produced by a cochlear implant.

However, research over the past decade has shown the benefit of treating single-sided deafness with cochlear implants. In 2019, the FDA approved for the first time the use of a cochlear implant to treat this form of hearing loss.

Single-sided deafness can arise from several causes, including tumors, head trauma, bacterial and viral infections, and structural problems in the ear. Or the trigger may not be known. This form of hearing loss creates an imbalance in hearing that makes it difficult to understand what is being said if there's background noise, as well as to determine what direction sounds are coming from. Many people with single-sided deafness also experience tinnitus or perceived ringing or other noises in the ear.

Understandably, single-sided deafness can be challenging and upsetting, leading to social isolation and reduced quality of life. In children, single-sided deafness can affect development and make children more likely to have trouble in school and need academic intervention.

Traditionally, treatment options have included special hearing aid systems that use microphones that reroute sound from the affected ear to the hearing ear — a technique known as contralateral routing of signal (CROS) — and bone

A team of specialists is involved in the process. Surgery is generally performed by an otolaryngologist, known as an ear, nose and throat (ENT) doctor, or a neuro-otologist who has had training in ear surgery. (Not all otolaryngologists perform the procedure.)

Other team members generally include an audiologist, a speech-language pathol-ogist, an educational consultant and a psychologist.

Your doctor can refer you to a cochlear implant center for evaluation. These centers are located throughout the United States and in other countries. The testing at these centers may help you with the many issues you'll need to consider as you proceed with implantation.

conduction devices (BCDs), which direct signals to the hearing ear using vibrations. However, both of these have their drawbacks, including poor tolerance and lackluster hearing improvements in some people.

Recent research on the impact of cochlear implants in people with single-sided deafness found improvements in many different areas, including determining where sounds were coming from, speech understanding with background noise and quality of hearing. Also important to note is that there was no evidence that a typical hearing ear and an ear that has a cochlear implant couldn't work together.

Mental health aspects also improved when using an implant, including less tinnitus stress and less emotional and cognitive distress. Research found that people who had cochlear implants didn't avoid stressful situations and had better coping mechanisms.

Cochlear implants didn't help all people, however. Participants in some studies reported that their tinnitus symptoms had worsened. For those who did benefit from the implant, it's unknown how long these improvements lasted, as follow-up periods for studies were often short — typically about six months. More research is needed to see how long implants maintain improved hearing and if hearing continues to improve over the long term.

Before the procedure

Before cochlear implant surgery, you'll have a complete evaluation. You or the implant center can end this process at any time if it's not appropriate to continue. This evaluation will generally include the following.

Medical evaluation

The ENT doctor will examine the health and function of your ear (otological examination). This is done to ensure that you don't have an active infection or a condition that precludes the use of an implant. You may also have a general exam to make sure you can safely undergo general anesthesia.

Imaging tests

Your doctor will review X-rays, CT scans and MRI of your inner ear. These tests show the condition of your cochlea, auditory nerve and inner ear. The health and structure of your ear play a significant role in how well a cochlear implant will work.

Audiological evaluation

An audiologist performs an extensive series of hearing tests to determine how well you can hear with and without appropriately adjusted hearing aids. The audiologist will also help you understand the benefits and limitations of a cochlear implant.

Balance exam

Because the hearing and balance systems are so closely connected, you may undergo testing to assess your balance. With cochlear implant surgery, there's a risk that one of your balance centers may be affected.

Speech and language evaluation

Standard speech and language tests are done to assess how well you use and understand language. A baseline, determined before surgery, gives your doctor information to compare against after surgery to see how well the cochlear implants are working for you.

Mental health evaluation

You may have tests to assess your ability to learn to use cochlear implants and how well you'll cope with lifestyle changes following the procedure.

If the results from these evaluations indicate that you're a candidate for implantation, you'll be scheduled for surgery. You and your surgeon will determine which ear would be best for the implant.

The surgeon may recommend bilateral implants as your best option. It's becoming more common to implant devices in both ears of children and some adults. There's evidence that two implants help users identify the source of sounds and improve understanding of speech.

Before surgery, your implant team will talk to you about the benefits and limitations of a cochlear implant, care and use of the device, the surgery itself, and post-surgical follow-up. If you or a family member feels anxious during this process, feel free to ask questions and express your concerns.

While cochlear implant surgery is generally safe, it does carry some risks:
- Loss of residual hearing. A cochlear implant may cause you to lose any remaining, unclear, natural hearing.
- Inflammation of the membranes surrounding the brain and spinal cord (meningitis). Vaccinations to reduce the risk of meningitis are generally given to adults and children before surgery.
- Failure of the device. You may need surgery to repair or replace the device if it fails to work.

Surgery

Cochlear implant surgery is performed under general anesthesia and lasts between two and four hours. You may have the procedure done as an outpatient, with no hospital stay.

After you're given medication to put you in a sleep-like state (anesthesia), the surgeon makes an incision behind the ear and exposes the mastoid bone. A small hole is created in the bone. This is where the internal device is placed.

A small opening is made in the cochlea, and tiny wires with the electrodes are inserted. Other times, the surgeon inserts the electrodes through a natural opening called the round window. Electronic tests are performed to make sure the stimulator is functioning properly with the intact nerve fibers. Then the incision is closed.

When you wake up from anesthesia, you'll have a bandage wrapped around your head. This will help reduce swelling around the incision.

You may experience some pain and nausea, but you can take medications for both forms of discomfort. On the day of surgery, most people are able to get out of bed for short walks.

A day or two after surgery, the head bandage will be removed. Your doctor will give you instructions as to what to do — and not to do — to take care of your incision as it heals.

Complications of cochlear implant surgery are rare. Some people say they have a bitter or metallic taste in their mouth or other differences in their sense of taste right after surgery. But typically, this eventually goes away.

Because the surgery involves your inner ear, your system of balance may be disrupted. This can cause dizziness or vertigo, which usually improves over the first 3 to 4 days, followed by a period of mild unsteadiness for a few weeks. By gently increasing activity, even though you may be slightly dizzy, your balance should gradually return to how it was before surgery.

The nerve controlling facial expressions runs through the surgical area. Rarely, this nerve may be weakened after surgery due to temporary swelling. You may notice that your smile isn't quite straight or you have trouble closing an eyelid. If this happens, it usually happens within the first two weeks after surgery. This may be short-term or long-term; your doctor can discuss options for treatment with you.

It takes up to four weeks after surgery for the incision to heal. Most people who receive cochlear implants resume regular activity within a few days to two weeks after surgery. Once the incision heals, the implant is noticeable on the outside only as a slight bump to the touch.

Activation

A cochlear implant is inactive when it's implanted and while you're healing. Deciding when to activate the device is the next step in the process.

Most centers wait a few weeks to a month before activating a cochlear implant. This allows time for the incision to heal and for you to recover from the anesthesia.

CARE AND HANDLING

Members of your cochlear implant team will provide detailed instructions for taking care of your implant's external components. These tips also may help:

- Try to avoid extreme heat and conditions that could cause breakage.
- Remove external components before participating in activities that generate high levels of static electricity, such as using trampolines or plastic slides. Like other electronic devices, the speech processor can be damaged by static electricity.
- You can wear the implant while participating in most sports. While it doesn't require extraordinary precautions, it's always a good idea to wear protective headgear for activities for which a helmet is recommended, such as bicycling, in-line skating, football and skiing.
- Turn off the speech processor before changing batteries, replacing cords or plugging something into it.
- Don't store batteries in the refrigerator. Putting a cold battery in a processor may cause condensation problems.
- Keep the microphone and processor in an anti-humidity kit when not in use. This is sometimes called a dryer or dry-aid kit.
- Most current controllers and processors are either water-resistant or waterproof. Depending on the processor, it may not be necessary to remove the external components before participating in water activities. Confirm with your implant team what to do when bathing or swimming.

You'll then meet several times with the audiologist to complete the process of fitting the external components and programming (mapping) the sound processor.

For some adults, activation soon after surgery may be an option. But at the same time, early activation may be somewhat uncomfortable and programming the device less precise.

Typically, at your first programming session with the audiologist, the headset or sound processor containing the microphone is placed on your head. The processor is connected to the audiologist's computer and programming equipment. The transmitter also is positioned, held in place by a magnet that couples with the magnet in the implanted receiver.

The amount of electrical stimulation required for a hearing response will then be determined for some or all of the electrodes. You'll be asked to respond each time you hear a sound and to signal when the loudness of each sound is most comfortable.

The audiologist will feed the information you provide into special computer software that programs your sound processor. The sound processor is set to certain levels of stimulation for each electrode, based on your responses to the sounds.

After the programming is complete, the processor is disconnected from the audiologist's computer. Batteries are inserted into the processor, and you're able to take the system home.

Your audiologist will schedule more visits to fine-tune the processor. Repeated adjustments are necessary because it takes time for your auditory nerve to adapt to the signals from the electrodes and for your brain to interpret these signals.

Complete programming varies. During the first year of use, the processor is reprogrammed often — you may have six or more appointments. Fewer visits are required after that. Experienced users usually visit just once a year.

Adjusting to an implant

Everyone who receives a cochlear implant has a different experience. Some people quickly appreciate sounds they haven't heard for many years. Other users need a gradual period of adjustment.

The sounds you first hear with a cochlear implant may seem unnatural. Often, speech will be unclear and hard to understand. With time, these sounds become more familiar as your brain relearns how to hear with the implant.

The process of adjustment is often slow and can take anywhere from weeks to years. Users who haven't had a long period of hearing loss can often understand speech rather quickly without speech reading. Users who have never had hearing before often need a longer time to adjust to the sounds.

SCOTT'S STORY: 'IT'S THE BEST THING I EVER DID'

Scott was born with hearing impairment, and it gradually got worse throughout his life. In grade school, he started experimenting with hearing aids, but they didn't help. Scott had difficulty recognizing and understanding what was being said, known as speech discrimination.

Although Scott became a self-described expert lip reader and felt like he was getting by with his hearing loss, it posed many challenges. Communicating with family wasn't easy, and Scott found himself in difficult situations when he didn't hear something correctly.

After many years of testing, Scott was approved to receive a cochlear implant. But he didn't jump at the chance right away. After years of coping with hearing loss, he felt like life was OK until someone asked him a question that made him reconsider: "Don't you ever wonder what's going on the other side of this closed door?"

Scott went ahead with cochlear implant surgery, and it was a success. Everything went smoothly, and Scott didn't have any complications.

Next came a new challenge: learning to hear.

"Probably the hardest thing about learning to hear again is that everything has to be mapped," Scott says. "Every new sound that you hear that you have never heard before, you have to learn it. You hear the sound but you've got to understand what the sound is."

For example, one day while Scott was in his kitchen, he heard a sound he didn't recognize. As it turns out, it was his dog drinking water from a bowl. Day by day, Scott's been amassing an entire library of sounds, learning them one by one and storing them in his brain so he knows what they are the next time he hears them.

Looking back on his years of not hearing well, Scott has no regrets about moving forward with cochlear implant surgery.

"It's the best thing I ever did," Scott says.

Learning to listen and make sense of sound requires dedicated effort. It also requires consistent exposure to sound. Adjusting to a cochlear implant will be easier — and you'll gain greater benefit — if you wear the device full time.

Start out with easier listening situations, like a conversation with one person in a quiet setting. With time, work up to more challenging situations, like group conversations or listening in places with lots of background noise. Also practice listening to the radio and television.

Adult users can benefit from various support services. Working with an audiologist, speech-language pathologist or teacher of people with hearing impairment, you can practice identifying sounds, recognizing speech and using speech reading. Speech training can help you speak more clearly and with good voice quality.

Your training may include listening-only activities and practice with a telephone. You may be given instructions on how to continue auditory training at home. Many web-based training programs are available over the internet for free or at a marginal cost.

Rehabilitation training and education are essential for children who receive a cochlear implant. It's only with training that a child will get the full benefit of the device. A child must learn to associate meanings to all of the new, unfamiliar sounds. Children must also be taught to understand the sounds and integrate them into language.

Speech-language pathologists, educators and family members can help reinforce the skills that your child is learning. The process takes time, dedication and a lot of hard work. But training throughout childhood usually leads to continuous improvements in performance.

Additionally, your audiologist or speech-language pathologist may provide other strategies to improve communication and handle difficult listening situations (see Chapter 8).

STAY POSITIVE

Cochlear implants are devices that can help you hear more easily. In turn, they may help you more fully take part in activities that require clear hearing.

If you choose a cochlear implant, know that much of your success is up to you. Before surgery, make sure you understand how much time you'll need to spend working with the implant. Talk to your care team about any questions you have. Using your implant as much as you can, making it to all of your follow-up visits and doing the listening exercises you're given will boost your odds for success.

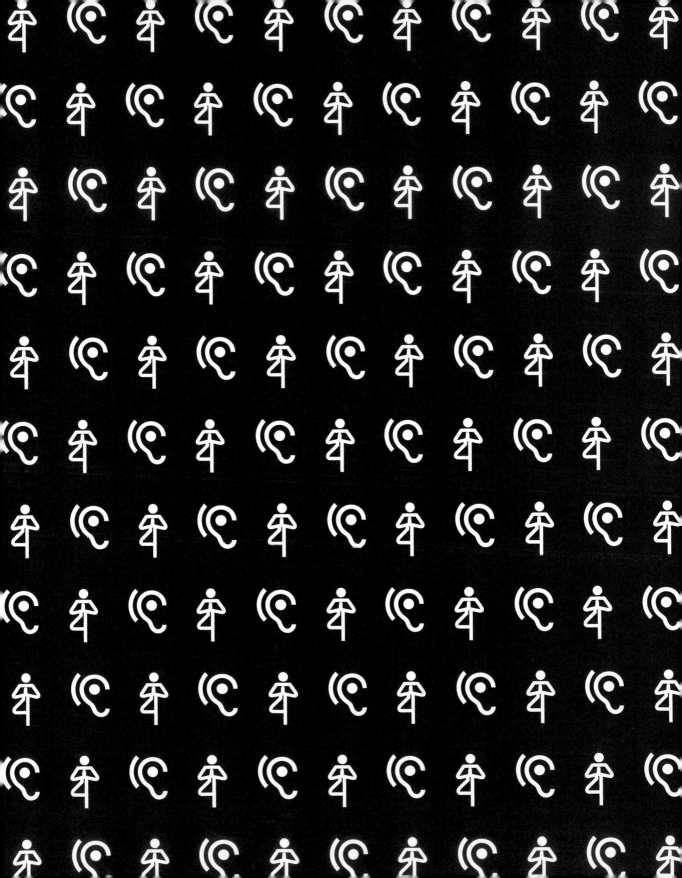

Other options to communicate better

11

Hearing aids and cochlear implants are valuable tools if you have a hearing impairment. But other options, including special listening devices, wireless technology and even your cellphone, can help you in many challenging situations.

These technologies can resolve common problems you face every day and make your life easier and safer. They can alert you to a doorbell ring, allow you to listen to a TV at a reasonable volume, and make it possible to talk by phone. They also make it easier to take part in public events and activities.

Communication technologies aren't meant to replace hearing aids or cochlear implants. Instead, they support these devices and enhance your hearing in difficult listening environments. Noisy

restaurants and lecture halls where sound reverberates are examples. These technologies allow you to lead a more independent and flexible lifestyle.

Devices are especially useful when you aren't wearing your hearing aids, like when you're in bed or in the shower. These devices can alert you to sounds you need to be aware of, like an alarm clock, smoke alarm or security alarm.

A variety of devices and services are available to use at home and in public places. Offices, restaurants, hospitals, churches and other public places provide information on the hearing services they offer on their websites and on site.

Under the Americans with Disabilities Act (ADA) and other legislation, public places are required to make reasonable accommodation for people who are deaf or have hearing loss.

What "reasonable" means can vary but may include assistive listening devices, captioning services and alerting technology. Find workplace-specific accommodations in Chapter 8.

WHY USE ASSISTIVE LISTENING DEVICES?

Many situations in daily life can disrupt your ability to hear and to function effectively. Three factors are often involved, either alone or in combination, to cause the problem: noise, distance and reverberation.

Noise

The hum of an air-ventilation system, traffic sounds or the scraping of chairs on the floor may keep you from understanding what's being said. Add to that the competing background noise of other people speaking, such as in a crowd or restaurant, and hearing becomes even more challenging.

Distance

It becomes harder to hear the farther away you are from the speaker — or the farther off to the side you are from the speaker. The best distance for hearing speech is between 3 and 6 feet. Even with hearing aids, these factors can make

hearing difficult. Environments that pose the most challenges include:

- Places with a lot of commotion and background noise, such as restaurants, cafeterias, lobbies, malls, subways and airports. An office can be a noisy place with the sound of foot traffic, conversation, manufacturing equipment, printers, copiers, telephones and radio.
- Situations where several people are talking at once, such as parties and social gatherings.
- Large rooms and facilities where a speaker may be far away, such as places of worship, classrooms, theaters and stadiums.
- Locations where sound waves echo, such as classrooms, hallways, basements, open offices, worship halls, arenas and warehouses.
- Situations where a steady, constant background noise is created by a fan, air conditioner, traffic or wind. This type of noise includes travel noise from highways or rails when you're riding in a car or a train.
- Outdoor activities where sound waves are dispersed, such as sporting events, festivals, parades and barbecues.
- Telephone conversations, especially when the connection isn't clear. These conversations are especially difficult because you can't use visual cues to improve your understanding.

Reverberation

Confined areas with hard surfaces, concrete block walls or uncarpeted floors are likely to echo sounds. Because these surfaces reflect sound waves multiple times, sound persists even after the sound source is cut off. This reverberation makes hearing difficult.

Many of these environments are difficult to avoid and hard to anticipate. Yet circumstances often require you to participate in them as you go about your daily life. Technology developed for these situations can help you function effectively in these environments.

Assistive listening devices (ALDs) are designed to improve your ability to hear in situations where conventional hearing aids aren't enough. ALDs are useful for many social, educational, occupational and entertainment activities, as well as for personal use at home.

HOW ASSISTIVE LISTENING DEVICES WORK

Assistive listening devices can help you in noisy rooms and in group conversations. They make it easier to use a telephone. In addition, ALDs may be used in one-on-one conversations with a friend and for listening to television or radio while you're relaxing alone. They can also be useful in the workplace during group meetings.

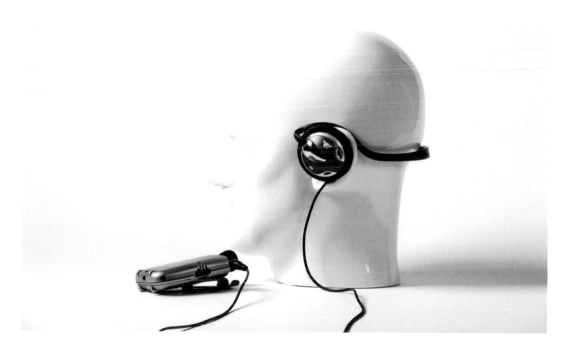

Personal amplifiers are a type of ALD used to increase volume in face-to-face and small-group conversations. The small boxes have both a microphone and listening cord connected to them. Both talker and listener share the same device.

Several ALDs are designed for use in large rooms, where people with hearing loss may have trouble understanding a distant speaker at a podium or on a stage. Frequently, in these settings listeners face problems not only because of distance from the speaker but also because of reverberation and background noise.

In classrooms, teachers often move from side to side or turn away from the class, so the volume of their speech fluctuates. In these situations, asking the teacher to talk louder may not solve your problems. Turning up the volume makes it easier to hear, but it may not make speech easier to understand.

ALDs make the sound or signal that you want to hear stand out from noises you don't. The signal might be a faraway voice coming over a static-filled telephone line, or a friend's voice that gets lost in the clatter of a noisy restaurant.

Although ALDs can usually amplify sounds, their primary purpose isn't to make sounds louder. Rather, they place a microphone close to the source of the sound you want to hear so that the sound is clearer and louder than other sounds in your environment.

ALD systems are equipped with different microphones, headphones and other features, but all systems are based on two components: a transmitter and a receiver. The transmitter, located close to the person speaking, picks up the sounds and converts them to signals, then broadcasts the signals. Often, there's a direct hookup to a microphone.

The receiver, located close to a listener, picks up the signals and introduces them to the listener's ears. Receivers carried by different individuals in the same audience can pick up the same signal from a single transmitter.

BUYING ALDS AND OTHER COMMUNICATION AIDS

Many assistive listening devices (ALDs) are provided free of charge in public places. If you're planning to buy an ALD or another form of communication aid for personal use, discuss the different options with your audiologist. Various devices may be on display at a local audiological center or speech, language and hearing center, university, or community agency. Websites also offer a wide selection of products with in-depth information.

These devices vary in price, so it's wise to comparison shop and work with someone who's knowledgeable about the technology. Check the warranty and return policy before you buy — some products come with as much as a five-year warranty. The staff who dispenses ALDs should provide you with training, including how to check and recharge batteries.

Some ALDs are designed for use with hearing aids or cochlear implants. Many that are used with hearing aids require that the aid have a feature such as a telecoil (T-coil), telephone switch, hookup (port) for direct audio input or built-in Bluetooth compatibility.

TELEPHONE DEVICES

Using the telephone can be a special challenge. For one thing, a conventional telephone doesn't amplify sound loud enough for individuals with hearing loss. For another thing, the listener can't see the speaker. This means there are no visual cues to help with understanding.

This is where a telephone amplifier can be useful. It's one of the most common ALDs, and it can be used with a cellphone or with a wired, cordless or digital phone. An amplifier allows you to adjust the volume of incoming calls so that even soft voices can be heard. Someone with no hearing loss can easily use the device, too.

Many new telephones come directly from the manufacturer with a built-in amplifier. An amplifier may be installed in the telephone body or in the handset when

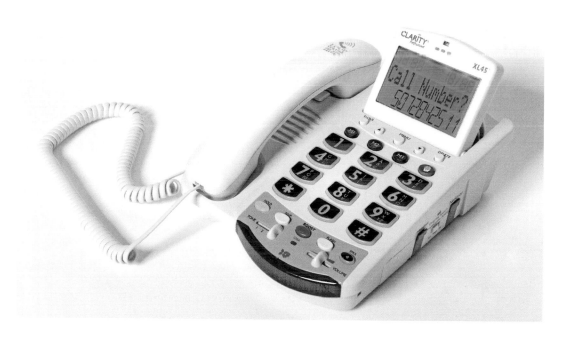

The controls at the bottom of an amplified telephone's body allow you to adjust the volume to your preference. A decal on the phone receiver indicates that this phone can amplify a speaker's voice.

If you have severe or profound hearing loss, using text-to-voice or captioned forms of TRS with a communications assistant requires that you have a special telephone with a display screen for text.

A captioned telephone allows you to hear the caller's voice and simultaneously see what's being said. The captions entered by a communications assistant appear on your telephone's display screen. You place a call in the same way that you would on a standard telephone, and you're automatically connected to the captioning service.

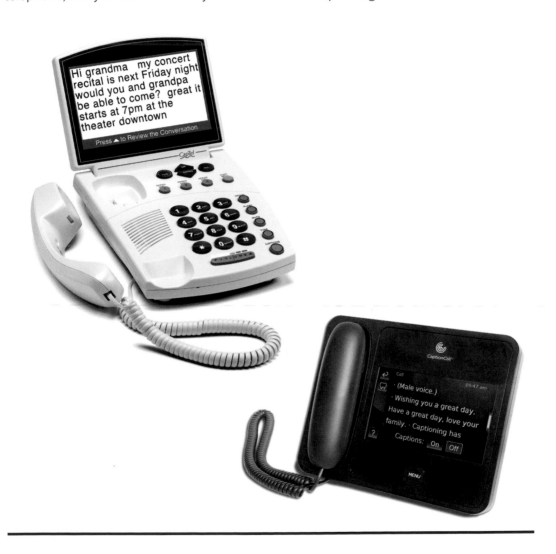

the mouthpiece, receiver and buttons are included as one unit. An amplifier may also be added as an in-line unit between the telephone and the wall jack.

Amplifier handsets may be installed in some public telephones, particularly at airports, train stations, museums and galleries, and hotel lobbies. A special telephone access sign on the receiver will identify whether amplification service is available.

Portable, snap-on amplifiers are small, battery-operated devices that can be carried with you in a purse or briefcase. When you're in situations where it's unlikely that you'll find a phone with an amplifier handset, you can slip the device over the receiver of most telephones. These portable amplifiers are especially helpful when you're traveling or when you're on the go.

Also portable, telephone adapters work with the telecoil in your hearing aids or cochlear implants. The adapter doesn't amplify sound but instead generates an electromagnetic field in response to sound waves. This allows the telecoil to pick up the sound directly. An adapter may work with some phones that aren't compatible with portable amplifiers.

When purchasing a new phone, be sure to verify with the supplier if the phone is compatible with a telecoil or portable amplifier.

Some telephones have special ringers that produce either an extra-loud ring or variable rings. Call indicators use a flashing light to inform you of incoming calls. Speakerphones can be useful in certain situations because they allow a person with hearing loss to listen with both ears.

Telecommunications Relay Service

People with severely limited hearing or no hearing at all can't use a standard telephone, even with an amplifier or adapter. They can still communicate over phone lines, however, by using a Telecommunications Relay Service (TRS).

TRS is a public service that costs nothing for its users. That's because the Americans with Disabilities Act requires U.S. telephone companies to provide the service free throughout the country. The phone companies are compensated with either state or federal funds. All services are available in English, but other languages, like Spanish and French, are available.

Using TRS requires someone with hearing loss to have a special phone that's equipped with a keyboard and text display monitor — a telecommunications device for the deaf (TDD) — or a captioned telephone (see page 192). Certain types of relay services can also function with a personal computer.

TRS provides real-time communication by adding a third-party operator, called a communications assistant (CA), into your phone conversation. The CAs are on call 24 hours a day at TRS relay centers located throughout the country.

You provide the CA with the telephone number to be called, either by speaking it into the handset or by typing and sending it via the keyboard. The CA places the call and then relays the spoken and written messages back and forth between you and the person you are calling.

The CA quickly converts spoken or written words into either text or voice. CAs are trained to be unobtrusive and to relay your conversations exactly as they're received. All calls through TRS are strictly confidential.

The Telecommunications Relay Service is easy to use. Anyone can use this service by calling 711 — the number that the federal government has reserved for access to TRS. Callers pay only the standard cost of a phone call. For many years, people with hearing loss have also used a text telephone device (TTY or TDD machine) to access this service.

There are several forms of TRS to consider, depending on your hearing loss and your personal preference:

Text to voice

This is the standard method of TRS service, with a CA serving as an intermediary between the spoken and written portions of the phone conversation. The CA speaks what a text user types and types what a voice telephone user speaks.

A voice-carry-over (VCO) option allows a person with hearing loss to speak directly to the other person. The CA types the

response. Similarly, with hearing carry over (HCO) a person with speech impairment can still hear the other party's voice and then relay a typed response through the CA.

Captioned service

This form of TRS uses voice recognition technology to convert the CA's spoken voice into written text. The captions are transmitted directly to a text display screen on your telephone.

Internet protocol (IP) relay service

With this internet-based form of TRS, a call goes from your computer to an IP relay center, which is usually accessed from a webpage. The CA relays your message via spoken voice over the regular telephone network.

You don't have to have a text or captioned telephone to use this service. A computer or any other web-enabled device such as a cellphone will do. The service connects directly to many forms of instant messaging and wireless text messaging programs.

IP captioned telephone service combines the internet-based system with a captioned telephone display. You speak directly to the called party and can listen to the response. At the same time, the CA repeats what's being said and speech recognition technology allows you to see the words almost instantly on your computer display.

Video relay service (VRS)

Another internet-based form of TRS is a bridge between individuals using sign language and individuals using spoken English. A CA communicates with the sign language user via a computer or tablet monitor and video equipment. Not all state TRS programs offer this service.

With the advent of modern communication devices, TTY machines are nearly a thing of the past. Instead, people often place calls using any device with a keypad or on-screen keyboard, such as a laptop, personal digital assistant or cellphone. With as popular as text messaging has become, many opt to skip the Telecommunications Relay Service entirely.

In addition to text messaging, many social media applications offer the ability for messaging. Social media accounts are typically free to set up and can be accessed through cellphones, computers or tablets, making them widely accessible to many individuals.

Multipurpose communication devices

Advances in computer hardware and electronics continue to create smaller and more-adaptable devices. This helps make many communication aids more portable, flexible and convenient.

Single devices have been developed that combine multiple functions. For example, a device that may look and function as a hearing aid — when needed — is also capable of other functions, serving as your wireless telephone with access to the internet, voicemail and more.

Wireless technology takes these developments a step further. Wireless networks use low-power radio waves to link computers and other devices together — no wires or cable hookups are required for them to communicate. Generally, the units must be located close together.

Bluetooth technology can connect as many as eight different devices together at the same time. That means — so long as all the devices are Bluetooth-enabled -- your hearing aid, computer, telephone and music player can be interacting simultaneously.

ASSISTIVE LISTENING SYSTEMS

Assistive listening systems improve the sound quality and volume of public-address systems for people with hearing loss. In most public places, one of three systems is generally installed: frequency modulated (FM), infrared and induction loop.

Frequency modulated (FM) systems

At public speaking events, you may be seated far from and not directly in front of the speaker. The sound system may be poor quality, and the audience members may move about and talk among themselves. By using a special listening system, such as an FM system, you can hear the speaker more clearly even with these challenges.

You may be familiar with the letters *FM*, from tuning your radio to a specific frequency to hear your favorite music or talk show. FM systems transmit sounds via radio waves, just like a mini radio station. FM systems operate on special frequencies assigned by the Federal Communications Commission (FCC). FM systems are commonly installed in locations where large audiences gather, such as auditoriums, convention centers, places of worship and theaters.

An FM system consists of two main components: a transmitter and a receiver. The transmitter can broadcast anything from a microphone, radio, television or stereo. It sends an FM signal to a small portable receiver that is tuned to the correct FM frequency.

HEARING AIDS AND CELLPHONES

To make cellphones more accessible, the Federal Communications Commission (FCC) has set rules that make it easier for people to choose a cellphone that will work well with hearing aids and cochlear implants. To find a cellphone that works well with hearing aids, look for a rating of M3 or M4.

When you're shopping for a cellphone, also look for its T rating. This refers to how well the phone works when a hearing aid is set to telecoil. If you use a hearing aid or cochlear implant with a telecoil, look for a cellphone with a rating of T3 or T4.

When shopping for cellphones that are compatible with hearing aids, look for the ratings to appear in one of these places.
• On a card next to the display phone
• On the phone's package
• In the user manual

If these ratings aren't marked on the package, ask the service provider or the device manufacturer for the rating information. Most often, if you can't find this label, the phone isn't hearing aid compatible.

Other features you might want to consider in a cellphone include vibrating alerts or a flashing screen, text messaging services, TDD mode, speech-to-text and video streaming. Many cellphone stores will allow you try out a cellphone in the store before you buy it. Make sure you bring your hearing aids with you when purchasing a new cellphone. This will allow you to see which features are right for you.

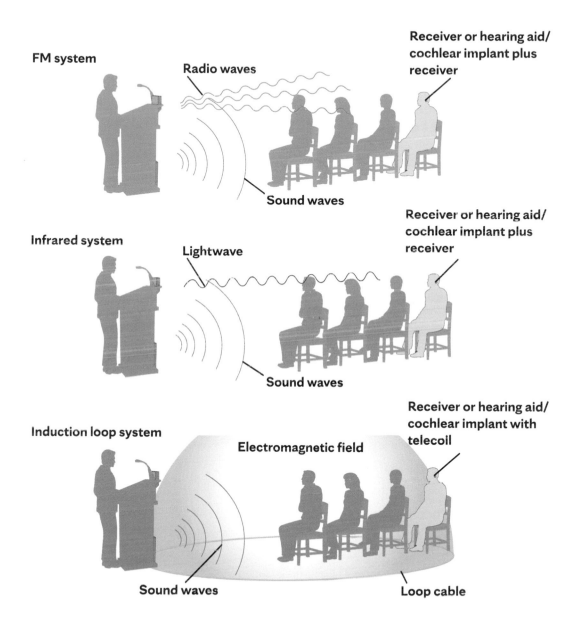

FM system

Radio waves

Receiver or hearing aid/
cochlear implant plus
receiver

Sound waves

Infrared system

Lightwave

Receiver or hearing aid/
cochlear implant plus
receiver

Sound waves

Induction loop system

Electromagnetic field

Receiver or hearing aid/
cochlear implant with
telecoil

Sound waves

Loop cable

Receivers come in several forms. Listeners can use a receiver that has volume control and converts the signal to sound via headphones. Another option is to have a receiver attached to a looped cord of wire (neck loop) that converts the FM signal into electromagnetic waves that are picked up by a telecoil in a hearing aid or cochlear implant.

Other receivers can be attached to a small adaptor (boot) that attaches to some behind-the-ear hearing aids or cochlear implants and sends the signal directly to the hearing aid or implant. This is known as direct audio input (DAI).

Personal FM systems can be used for one-on-one communication. Composed of a small, portable microphone, receiver and amplifier, they're useful for private conversations in difficult hearing environments such as noisy restaurants or highly reverberant auditoriums. As long as you're tuned to the correct frequency, you can use personal systems while you're walking or in a car, and you can use them to listen to television and radio stations.

A growing number of public buildings, government facilities and business offices are equipped with FM systems to accom-

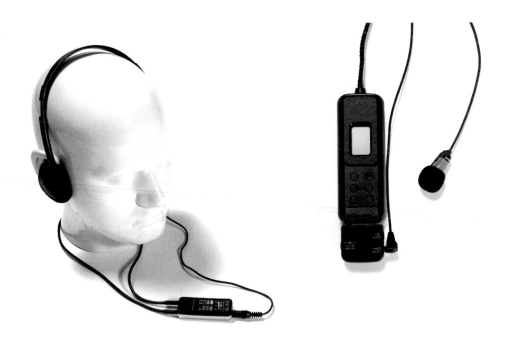

In a setting with a large audience, such as a classroom, an FM system with a transmitter and microphone (right) allows speakers to send their voices directly to you through a receiver that you wear with headphones (left) or hearing aids.

modate visitors with hearing loss. Many schools also are using FM technology to assist students with hearing impairment. A newer version of these systems, known as dynamic FM, further filters the signal and uses directional microphones to reduce noise, among other features.

Infrared systems

Some assistive listening systems use radio waves to carry sound. Others, like infrared systems, transmit sound via lightwaves to receivers worn by listeners with hearing loss.

Like FM systems, infrared systems are used in locations where hearing is difficult or in situations where large groups of people are gathered. Infrared technology is also commonly available for TV viewing at home.

When this system is used in a large auditorium, an infrared light emitter is plugged into an existing public-address system or sound system. The infrared lightwaves transmit speech or music to receivers that are worn by members of the audience. The receiver may be connected to headphones that introduce sound directly to the ear. Or the receiver

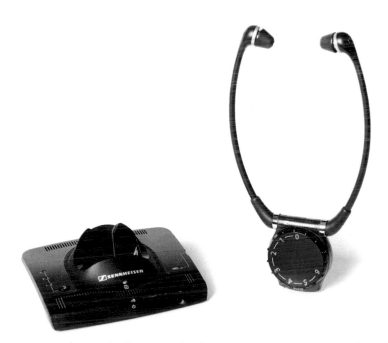

Infrared systems send sounds, for example, from a television program, directly to you from a unit that sits on the television (left). A lightweight headset that you wear (right) lets you adjust the device to a volume that you need for hearing while keeping the TV at a volume that's comfortable for others.

can be used with a neck loop linked to a hearing aid or cochlear implant equipped with a telecoil.

Using an infrared system with a television allows you to set the TV at a volume that's lower and more comfortable for other listeners. The infrared transmitter sends the TV signal to a personal receiver, which you can adjust as needed. But your adjustments don't affect the volume level heard by others in the room.

Unlike an FM system, an infrared system must have the receiver in the transmitter's direct line of broadcast to work well. Sunlight can interfere with the signal, so these systems aren't a good choice for outdoor use. In contrast, because infrared lightwaves are broadcast along a confined path and not emitted in all directions, infrared systems provide more privacy than FM systems do.

Infrared systems are often used in courtrooms and government offices and during live performances in theaters and auditoriums.

Induction loop systems

Induction loop systems, also called audio loop systems, transmit sounds using an

USING YOUR HEARING AID'S TELECOIL

Many behind-the-ear and in-the-ear hearing aids are equipped with a telecoil (T-coil). The telecoil is helpful for listening on the telephone. Typically, a hearing aid is sensitive to all sound waves. But when the telecoil is turned on, the aid amplifies only electromagnetic waves from the telephone's receiver. This means that the telephone signal is transmitted directly into the hearing aid without any other noise being amplified.

Most phones are compatible with hearing aids, but when you buy a phone, be sure to ask about hearing aid compatibility. If the salesperson doesn't know, try out the phone before buying it. A compatible unit should have an "HAC" label on its base. Find more information about hearing aid compliance and other standards for cellphones on page 196.

A telecoil can also be used with FM systems (see page 195) and induction loop systems (see this page).

Having a hearing aid with a telecoil broadens your communication options. If your hearing aid has a telecoil and you aren't sure how to use it, talk with your audiologist or hearing aid dealer for training.

electromagnetic field created by a loop of wire installed around the listening area. An amplifier and microphone transmit sound via an electric current that flows through the loop. Hearing aids and cochlear implants equipped with telecoils can receive these signals. Separate receivers can be provided to people who don't have the telecoil feature in their hearing aids or cochlear implants.

Induction loop systems can be permanently installed in the floors of auditoriums or chambers. Portable, temporary loop systems may be set up as needed.

Reception with induction loop systems is susceptible to electrical interference. Also, they're not as flexible as FM systems and infrared systems are for personal use.

Speech recognition systems

These systems allow you to capture voices with a microphone and convert what's being said into a visual display on a screen. They can use an external microphone or even the microphone in your cellphone. The visual display can be a computer, tablet or a cellphone. They can be very useful for someone with a hearing impairment.

Learning to use the software requires training and patience. In addition, it doesn't work well in tricky listening environments. For example, you can't walk into a noisy party, point the microphone in the direction of a speaker, and instantly read his or her words on a screen.

Visual communication systems

Visual communication technology is also helping people with hearing loss, especially those who use sign language as their primary means of communication. Video chat applications allow people to communicate in sign language over the phone lines or the internet.

In addition, mobile apps are available that interpret spoken and written English and translate it into sign language. Another system provides sign language by way of a computer that's fitted with a digital camera and on-call interpreters.

CAPTIONING

Until the early 1970s, many people with hearing loss weren't able to fully enjoy one of America's favorite pastimes – watching television. In 1972, for the first time, a national TV program — Julia Child's cooking show, *The French Chef* — was broadcast with captions that reflected the audio portion of the show.

Since that broadcast, captions have opened the world of television to people who are deaf or have hearing loss. Hundreds of hours of entertainment, news, public affairs and sports programming are captioned each week on network, public and cable TV and streaming services.

Similar to movie subtitles, television captions display dialogue as printed words on the screen. Unlike subtitles, captions also indicate sounds like applause, music and laughter. The text is carefully positioned on the screen to identify who is speaking. Captions are encoded as data within the television signal, ready for immediate broadcast.

You can tell if a specific program is closed-captioned when the letters CC appear on the screen, often within a television-shaped symbol. Another symbol shows a small TV screen with a tail at the bottom (see page 203). Subtitles are also available with many streaming services.

Other uses of captioning

Captioning is included on many movies on DVD and Blu-ray Disc and available via streaming services. It's also featured on many educational and training films. Captioning is also provided for many live events, like musical and theater performances, lectures, government proceedings, in-person and online meetings, and conferences. Museums and science centers may use captioning in shows, self-produced films and demonstrations.

Some movie theaters offer a captioning system called rear-window captioning. An adjustable transparent plastic panel attaches to the viewer's seat and reflects captions displayed on a panel positioned at the back of the theater.

ALERTING DEVICES

Assistive technology can alert you to many special sounds in your environment. Awareness of these sounds is important for your safety and to maintain your independent lifestyle. Sounds that can be signaled include a telephone ring, alarm clock buzz, kitchen timer beep, doorbell chime, a knock at the door, the cry of a baby, and the peal of a smoke alarm or security alarm.

Alerting devices may use one or more of three types of signals to inform you of the sound — a loud sound, a flashing light or a vibration.

For example, an alarm clock can be wired with a vibrating attachment that's placed under your pillow. At the selected hour, you're gently shaken awake. Another option is an attachment with a flashing light that's plugged into your regular alarm clock.

Devices like a vibrating pager, wristwatch or fitness tracker or even the vibration setting on a cellphone can alert you in response to a paging system, time setting or another type of notification, like an incoming email, phone call or text message.

Alerting systems can be simple or complex. Some multipurpose alarms can use a code to indicate different sounds — for example, a telephone ring might be one light flash, the doorbell three flashes and the smoke alarm a series of on-off flashes. Some systems can be wired for use in several rooms or for transferring from room to room. Special alerting devices can also be used in your vehicle. For example, a siren alert can let you know when an emergency vehicle is nearby.

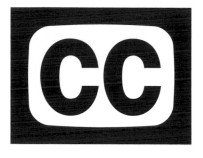 

Either of these symbols indicate that a television program is closed-captioned.

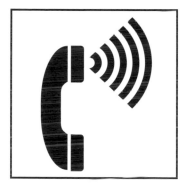

Amplified telephone

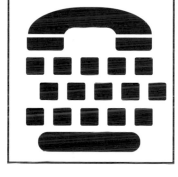

Text telephone

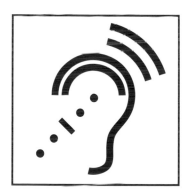

Assistive listening system

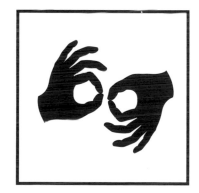

Sign language

When these international symbols appear in public buildings, it means services have been installed for individuals with hearing loss.

MANY OPTIONS ARE AVAILABLE

It wasn't long ago that hearing aids were just about the only communication aid available for people with hearing loss. Now, advances are bringing about new opportunities and major improvements to existing devices for people living with hearing loss. Researchers continue to search for new ways to improve lives.

Many people with hearing loss don't know about the many options in technology and computer software that can make communication easier. Assistive listening devices and other aids can make a significant difference in easing the daily problems caused by hearing loss. It's worthwhile to explore these options.

Of course, choosing among this ever-changing technology and knowing what might work best for you can be confusing at first. It's all too easy to be overwhelmed or seduced by the gadgetry.

If you're not sure where to start, talk to a hearing health professional, such as your audiologist or an ear, nose and throat specialist.

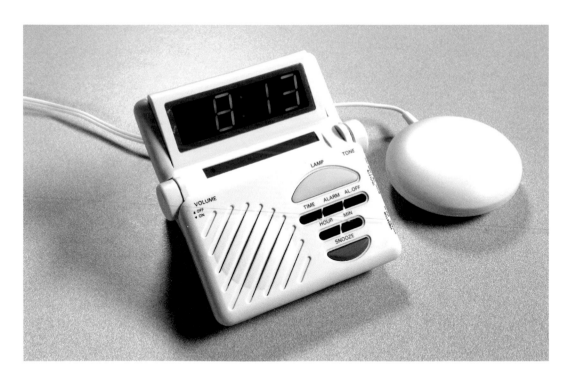

This alarm clock can employ any or all of three options to wake you: a loud sound, a flashing light and a vibrating attachment that can be placed under your pillow to gently shake you.

ASSISTIVE LISTENING DEVICES: NEXT STEPS

Write the listening situations most important to you below. Use examples in gray as a guide. Then talk with your audiologist about strategies that may help.

Place **Communication needs**

	Face to face	Media	Phone	Alerting
Home	One-on-one, group conversations	TV, computer, radio	Landline, cellphone	Doorbell, phone, alarm clock
Work	One-on-one, group conversations	TV, computer, radio	Meetings by phone or video	Fire alarms, knock at the door
Travel and leisure	Restaurants, cars, malls, tours	Movie theaters, concerts	Hotel phone, voicemail	Hotel alerts
School	One-on-one, group conversations, lectures in assembly halls	TV, computer, video	Landline, cellphone	Fire alarms, bells, timers

Adapted from: Alpiner JG, et al., eds. Assistive technology for enhancement of receptive communication. In: *Rehabilitative Audiology: Children and Adults*. 3rd ed. Lippincott Williams & Wilkins; 2000.

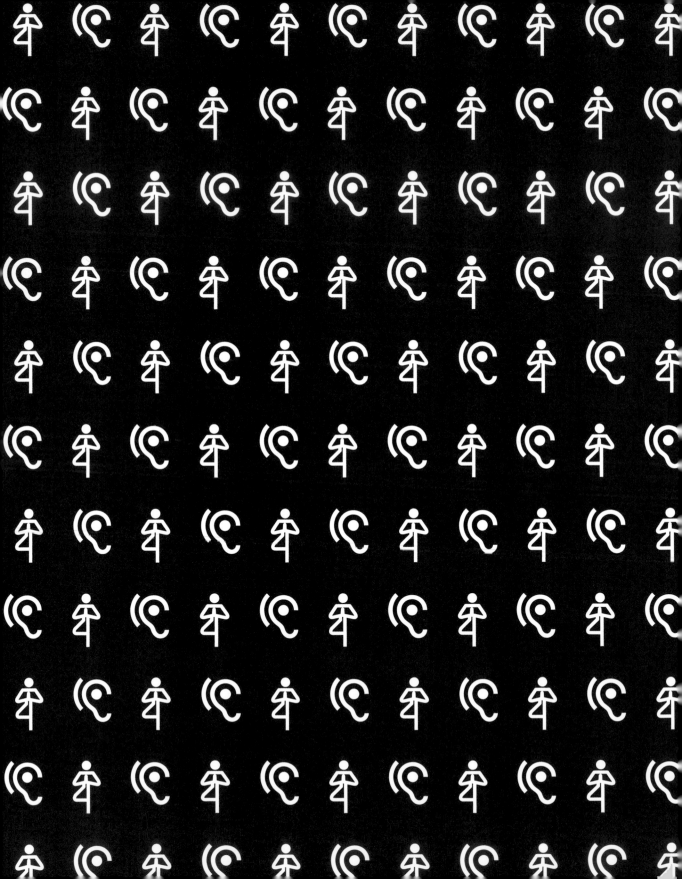

Kids and hearing health

12

Lexi was born profoundly deaf due to a hearing disorder known as auditory neuropathy. With this disorder, the inner ear detects sound but can't get sound signals to the brain. Because Lexi was having trouble hearing sound, she received her first cochlear implant when she was 4½ years old.

Although growing up with a hearing impairment can be challenging, it doesn't have to hold a child back from living fully and thriving. Lexi is proof positive of this. A college graduate, Lexi enjoys a fulfilling career. She also finds purpose by volunteering in her community and with organizations dedicated to supporting people with hearing impairments.

"I have no qualms in saying that if I wasn't deaf, I would not be the person I am

today. I am stronger and more confident than I would ever be if I had been born hearing," Lexi says. "I believe that a person's true character can be seen in how they respond to adversity. I have never let my disability define me and I try to set an example that there are no limitations to what I can achieve."

In this chapter, you'll learn about the tests done to support hearing health throughout childhood. You'll also learn about different types of hearing loss in children and how to help a child thrive with hearing loss.

REGULAR HEARING EXAMS

Newborn hearing screening is now a common practice in most hospitals in the

United States. That's because hearing loss is common, affecting up to 3 in every 1,000 children born in the U.S. each year. In most states, testing is required through Early Hearing Detection and Intervention (EHDI) programs. These programs ensure that all infants and young children with hearing loss are identified early and receive appropriate services. Failure to identify hearing loss early enough can lead to delayed speech and language development, social-emotional or behavioral problems, and learning delays.

Children with unidentified hearing loss often don't do as well in school as their peers do. They're also more likely to be held back a grade or drop out. Because hearing loss isn't always obvious, a child may mistakenly be seen as distracted or unmotivated. Early treatment can help prevent many problems related to hearing loss and provide a child with the tools needed to be successful at school.

Some types of hearing loss in children don't develop until months or years after birth. For this reason, periodic screening is recommended.

When do children get hearing tests?

Hearing tests are generally done throughout childhood at these points:

Infants and toddlers
- By 1 month of age: This is an initial screening, preferably done soon after birth.
- By 3 months of age: If the initial screening shows that a child may have hearing loss, more testing is done to confirm hearing loss.
- Before 6 months of age: Infants with hearing loss begin receiving treatment. Infants are monitored on ongoing basis.
- By 9 months of age: Children who passed their initial screening but have a risk factor for hearing loss have more testing. This testing may be needed more often for children at higher risk of hearing loss or when there are new concerns about hearing.

School-age children
- When entering the school system
- Every year from kindergarten through third grade
- At seventh grade
- At 11th grade
- When entering special education
- When repeating a grade
- When entering a new school system, if screening hasn't been done
- When indicated by parent or caregiver, by medical or school concern, or by high risk factors for hearing loss

In addition, babies considered to be at high risk of hearing loss should be screened regularly. This group includes babies who:
- Were born prematurely
- Experienced a severe lack of oxygen deprivation at or shortly after birth
- Were exposed to an infection in the womb, like German measles (rubella) or syphilis
- Were exposed to herpes when they passed through the birth canal
- Had meningitis
- Had severe jaundice
- Had head trauma

- Had a blood incompatibility with their mother
- Were born to a mother with diabetes
- Were born to a mother who used drugs or alcohol while pregnant
- Had a chronic ear infection
- Had any nervous system disorder associated with hearing loss
- Have a family history of childhood hearing loss
- Have inner ear problems like Mondini's malformation or enlarged vestibular aqueducts
- Had cytomegalovirus infection
- Had chemotherapy

Hearing tests for children

Objective tests can be used for children of all ages — including newborns — because the child can sleep or sit quietly through the tests. However, there also are many age-related behavioral approaches that audiologists can use for testing. Results are typically obtained by presenting various sounds through a combination of small earphones, bone conduction devices or sound field speakers.

There are five common types of hearing tests used most often for babies. Here's more on each of these types of tests, with details on how each one works.

Auditory brainstem response

This type of testing can be used at any age but is especially helpful for infants and young children. It involves placing small recording electrodes on the head and behind the ears. Different clicking sounds are played in the ears at different volumes and frequencies and the electrodes record the response coming from the hearing nerve.

Otoacoustic emissions

This type of testing can be used at any age, but it is most commonly used for infants and children. This test involves placing a small probe in the ear and playing a series of chirping sounds. The computer records the ear's response to those sounds.

Aside from auditory brainstem response and otoacoustic emissions testing, these three behavioral hearing tests are commonly used for children.

Behavioral observation audiometry

This type of testing is typically used for the youngest children, from newborns to babies up to 6 months old. It involves careful observation of changes in the child's behavior — such as eye widening, startling motions or changes in sucking behaviors — following the presentation of various sounds. Since children at this age can't respond reliably, this type of testing is interpreted with caution, along with the results of objective tests.

Visual reinforcement audiometry

This testing is commonly used for children from about 6 months through 2 years of age. Special animated lights and

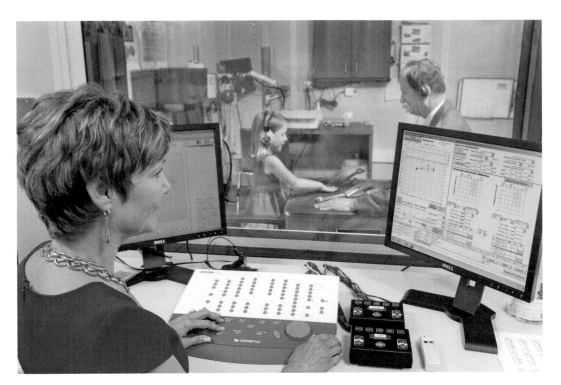

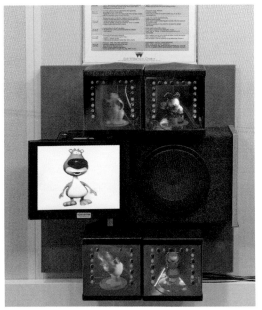

Conditioned play audiometry (above) tries to engage a child's response through play. As simple as they may seem, these play activities can reliably enable the audiologist to determine approximate hearing levels, often for each ear.

Visual reinforcement audiometry (left) incorporates special animated lights and toys to serve as "reinforcers" to a child's eye shifting or head turning in response to various types of sounds.

toys serve as "reinforcers" to a child's eye shifting or head turning in response to various types of sound. Sounds used may include the tester's voice or several low- and high-frequency signals.

Conditioned play audiometry

This testing is often used for children ages 2½ to 5 years old. It engages a child's response through play. Children may be asked to toss small blocks or toy figures into a bucket or pound the end of a small shovel loaded with plastic toys each time they hear a sound. While these activities may seem simple, they can reliably help the audiologist learn how well the child hears, often for each ear.

HEARING PROBLEMS AT BIRTH

Some hearing problems present at birth (congenital) run in families. Others develop in the womb or from conditions during the birthing process.

Hearing loss in children can take on many different forms and stem from many different causes. Some children are born with hearing loss, while others develop it later on. While the cause of hearing loss isn't always known, up to a quarter of hearing loss in babies can be traced back to environmental triggers, like an infection the mother had during pregnancy or complications after birth. But the most common cause of hearing loss is a genetic change (mutation), which causes hearing loss at birth or later in infancy or childhood. In some cases, a combination of genetic mutations and environmental triggers can cause hearing problems.

Genes are stored in DNA and are responsible for providing instructions that help cells function properly. If these genes are altered (mutated), it can cause problems with cell function and lead to health problems. Genetic mutations can be recessive, meaning two copies of the gene must be passed along to a child — one from each parent — for the child to be at risk of developing a condition. Mutations may also be dominant, meaning only one copy of an altered gene is needed to cause a condition or health problem in a child.

Genetic hearing loss is described as syndromic or nonsyndromic. In syndromic cases, hearing loss is part of a syndrome and one of many symptoms. For example, children born with Waardenburg's syndrome have hearing loss and irregularities in skin, eye and hair coloring. More than 400 genetic syndromes are known to cause hearing loss.

LEARN MORE

How do you know if your child might have hearing loss? Get tips from Mayo Clinic experts: links.mayoclinic.org/childhearing

The vast majority of children who have genetic hearing loss have a nonsyndromic form, which means it's not part of a larger syndrome. For these children, hearing loss is the only symptom.

Many genetic mutations exist that cause nonsyndromic hearing loss. The most common genetic mutations that cause nonsyndromic hearing loss are:

- A mutation in the GJB2 gene can cause severe to profound deafness. This gene is responsible for a protein called connexin 26, which aids in the functioning of the cochlea.
- A mutation in the STRC gene, which plays a role in making a protein called stereocilin, can cause mild to moderate hearing loss. Stereocilin assists with proper hair cell function in the ear.

AIDA'S STORY: 'A LITTLE MIRACLE'

Born prematurely, Aida failed her newborn hearing tests. After the second test, Aida's doctors shared with her parents the difficult news that Aida was deaf. The doctors explained that Waardenburg's syndrome — a rare genetic disorder that causes deafness and pigment changes in the hair, eyes and skin — was likely the cause.

"When you first hear it, you kind of say, 'That's not true,' or, 'What can we do to help it? You know, what can we do to make her hear?' I don't think I was ready for that kind of information," says Aida's mom, Melinda.

Among its many symptoms, Waardenburg's syndrome can cause changes in the inner ear that cause hearing impairment. According to some estimates, between 2% and 5% of cases of deafness at birth are caused by Waardenburg syndrome.

Because hearing aids didn't help Aida much, her parents turned to cochlear implants. Aida had cochlear implants placed in both ears when she was 7 months old.

Aida has adapted to the implants well, according to her parents. She wears a headband to hold the external processors in place, and she seems to understand its significance.

"She gets excited when she sees her headband come out in the morning," says Aida's mom, Melinda. "Putting on her sound changes everything; she becomes more animated and focused."

- Mutations in the TECTA gene, a gene that helps encourage the movement of the ear's sensory hair cells, can cause midfrequency hearing loss.

All of these genetic mutations tend to trigger hearing loss early in life or before a child would typically begin talking. Depending on the cause, hearing loss may be either progressive, which means it will worsen over time, or stable, meaning it won't get worse.

Newborn hearing screening can identify concern for hearing loss, usually before a baby leaves the hospital. However, the screening can't identify mutations or other causes. Genetic testing that uses DNA, such as a blood test, can look for mutations.

Aida works with a speech therapist, as well as a teacher from the Deaf community. She also goes to an audiologist regularly to have the cochlear implants reprogrammed, tuning each of their 22 channels to improve sound.

While there have been some challenges along the way — for example, sleeping alone in her bed without her cochlear implants on was scary for Aida at first — the family has worked together to help Aida work through her fears and to learn and understand the world around her.

Now 3 years old, Aida has experienced many successes with her cochlear implants. She knows how to put her implants on and how to put them back on if they fall off. She can use and understand spoken language well even when her implants aren't turned on. And she's starting to read lips — in fact, she can almost fully communicate vocally even when her cochlear implants are turned off. "We're all very, very shocked," Melinda says. "Typically when they're off, you lose that sense of how words are formed."

Being able to hear with cochlear implants has helped Aida socially, too. She can explain, in her own words, what cochlear implants are. And she can hear what other people hear, which enriches her relationships. For example, if her brother says he hears a bird chirping or a fire truck siren, Aida can hear it, too — and she lights up in excitement because she's sharing in the experience.

"Something so simple is huge for Aida," Melinda says. "She's such a little miracle."

Identifying a genetic cause helps health care providers predict how an inherited condition might progress and whether any other symptoms might appear. This can help a parent anticipate what to expect as a child grows and develops.

It's important to note that testing has limitations. For example, not all genes that cause hearing problems are known, so genetic testing may not uncover the cause. In other cases, it may be difficult to tell whether a mutation is causing a condition or just happens to be present.

As you learned earlier, most newborns are screened for hearing loss before they leave the hospital. Even when a baby receives passing results, it's important to continue monitoring the child's hearing as he or she develops. Screening helps identify problems with hearing. A hearing impairment, once identified, may then be successfully managed with hearing aids or cochlear implants. Treating hearing loss is critical for a child's speech and language development.

ACQUIRED HEARING LOSS IN CHILDREN

While many hearing problems can be present at birth, some develop later in childhood. At least 1 in 5 children with hearing loss acquired it after birth. Screening helps spot hearing loss so it can be treated.

Children may acquire hearing loss at any time as a result of a disease, condition or injury. Noise exposure is becoming a more common cause of acquired hearing

loss in children. Acquired hearing loss may be caused by:

- Noise exposure
- Ear infections
- Drugs that damage the hearing system (ototoxic)
- Meningitis
- Measles
- Encephalitis
- Chicken pox
- Influenza
- Mumps
- Head injury

More children are acquiring hearing loss because of noise. Studies show that more than 1 in 10 children and teenagers have hearing loss caused by noise. It's important to talk with your child about what noises are too loud and when to wear hearing protection. (Learn more in Chapter 4.) Volume limiters, available on most portable electronic devices, also can help prevent noise-induced hearing loss.

SUPPORT FOR CHILDREN WITH HEARING LOSS

Diagnosing and treating hearing loss as early as possible is critical. Prompt and successful treatment will help with a child's overall health, performance in school, language use, thinking and decision-making, self-esteem, and relationships with others. The sooner a child is treated for hearing loss, the more effectively the child will adjust and thrive.

Many support options are available for families and children with hearing loss. Ask your audiologist what resources are available in your state. The Individuals with Disabilities Education Act (IDEA) ensures that children with hearing loss receive intervention and education from birth through age 21.

The many tips, techniques and technologies you've read about in previous chapters can all help a child live well with hearing loss. In addition, parents can use certain skills alongside hearing aids and implants to further boost language use and understanding.

Language-building programs are family focused. Programs used with children include:

- **American Sign Language:** Teaches babies and young children to use a visual language system.
- **Auditory-oral:** Teaches babies and young children to use the hearing they have. Also uses lip-reading and gestures.
- **Auditory-verbal:** Teaches babies and young children who use cochlear implants to listen, to understand spoken language and to speak.
- **Bilingual:** Teaches babies and young children American Sign Language and the family's native language.
- **Cued speech (building block):** Helps children understand spoken languages.
- **Total communication:** Teaches babies and young children to use a combination of techniques to communicate in English. May use speech and signing at the same time.

In addition, as with adults, many other approaches are helpful with children. Limiting background noise and speaking clearly — as well as face-to-face — are all examples. Assistive listening devices like television listeners also may be helpful.

With the help and support of a team of professionals, parents may choose one or several of these programs to help their child communicate. The key is to find the best blend of devices, therapy and approaches that will help your child succeed. Look to your child's medical team, as well as community and school resources, to create the best plan for your child.

PART 5

Balance 101

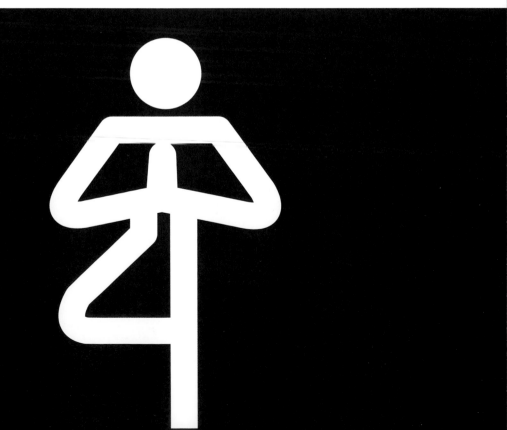

13

Getting a balance exam

The word *dizzy* is used to describe a variety of sensations — a false sense of motion, lightheadedness, weakness, loss of balance, faintness, wooziness and unsteadiness on your feet. You may feel that your surroundings are spinning around you — a condition commonly called vertigo.

There are many causes of dizziness, which disrupt the complex system of balance in your body. A critical element of this system is the vestibular labyrinth, the main balance organ that — together with the cochlea — is contained in your inner ear. Certain disorders of the inner ear, as you learned, can cause both hearing loss and dizziness.

Dizziness and vertigo — the sensation that your surroundings are whirling or spinning — are commonly associated with vestibular disorders. If you have a vestibular disorder, you may also experience nausea or vomiting, changes in heart rate and blood pressure, fear, anxiety, and even panic. These effects may make you feel tired, depressed and lacking focus.

Doctors often can determine the cause of dizziness, and for most people, the signs and symptoms last a short time. Even when no definite cause is found or in cases where the dizziness persists, your doctor can prescribe treatments that usually ease symptoms to a manageable level.

In this chapter, you'll discover how the body works to maintain balance and what tests are often done when you're having balance issues.

KEEPING YOURSELF BALANCED

Your balance system allows you to remain upright as you walk and move around or change position. It helps keep your vision focused and clear while your head is turning. Good balance also keeps you aware of the position of your head in relation to the ground.

To maintain your balance, your brain must coordinate sensory information from your eyes, your inner ear, the bottoms of your feet, and major joints such as the ankles, knees and neck. Then the brain tells the muscles in your body how to react and maintain your position.

This same information helps form your perceptions of how you're oriented in space, what direction you're moving in and how fast you're moving. Here's more on how your balance system works.

Your eyes

No matter what position you're in — sitting, standing, lying down or moving — visual signals help you determine where your body is in space. When light hits your retina, it generates electrical impulses that are sent to your brain through the optic nerve.

Your brain interprets these signals as images. The brain uses the images to calculate, for example, how far your chair seat is above the ground, or how far away a car is that's moving in front of you, or how fast you're moving relative to someone walking beside you.

Your nervous system

Millions of nerve cells (neurons) are located in your skin, muscles and joints. When touch, pressure and movement stimulate these cells, they send electrical impulses to your brain about what your body is doing — for example, whether you're lying down on a soft mattress or climbing up a stepladder.

Information about the movement of your neck and your ankles is especially important for balance because it tells your brain which way your head is turned and how steady you are on the ground.

Your vestibular labyrinth

The vestibular labyrinth is your primary balance organ. The brain uses this inner ear organ to tell where your head is relative to gravitational space, and whether your head or body is changing its position.

Although you're probably not as aware of the vestibular labyrinth as you are of your eyes, your brain relies on its input for balance. This is especially true when information from the eyes, joints or bottoms of your feet is disrupted.

A complex system

Problems with dizziness and balance can arise anywhere within your sensory system. To maintain balance across a full range of daily activities, at least two of the system's elements must work well.

For example, you likely won't lose your balance if you close your eyes when you're in the shower. That's because signals from your inner ear and musculoskeletal nerves keep you upright. But if your central nervous system can't process the signals properly or if your vestibular labyrinth isn't functioning correctly, you may get dizzy and fall in the shower.

TESTS FOR BALANCE ISSUES

If you're experiencing episodes of dizziness often, or if they last for long periods of time or are severe, talk to your doctor. You may need to have several tests to assess the health of your inner ear and balance system. An audiologist usually performs these tests.

Test results can help show if one or both ears are affected and how well your inner ear, eyes, muscles and joints work together. Test results may also show if you may benefit from therapy.

You'll likely be asked to not consume alcohol or take certain sedatives or tranquilizers for 24 hours before testing.

YOUR SYSTEM OF BALANCE

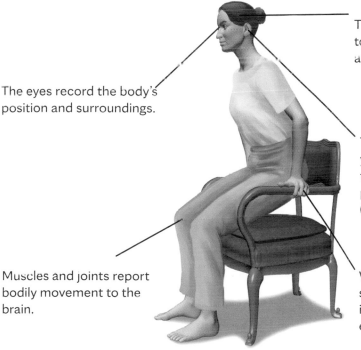

The brain relays information to and from the eyes, muscles and joints, skin, and inner ear.

The eyes record the body's position and surroundings.

The inner ear contains both your primary hearing structure (cochlea) and your primary balance structure (vestibular labyrinth).

Muscles and joints report bodily movement to the brain.

When you touch things, sensors in your skin give you information about your environment.

It's also recommended that you not eat within two hours of testing. You'll want to wear comfortable clothes, like sweatpants, for tests that require you to use a harness.

Most people find the tests to diagnose dizziness to be simple and nonthreatening. However, at times, they may make you feel dizzy, nauseous or anxious. Talk with your audiologist about any concerns before, during or after testing.

Your balance exam may include one or more of these tests.

Hearing test

Because the cochlea and vestibular labyrinth are both in the inner ear, problems with one of these structures often accompany issues with the other. For this reason, a hearing test is usually a common part of a balance exam. Get details about hearing tests in Chapter 7.

Nystagmography

Nystagmography is a series of tests that evaluate how your inner ear and eye

WHAT YOU SHOULD EXPECT

At your balance exam, you'll answer questions about your symptoms. You may also fill out a questionnaire to help describe the issues you're having. Your answers help determine what tests you'll have.

It's common to not know what to expect during balance tests. You may even worry that these tests will make you feel worse. You may find it reassuring to know that most people who have these tests say that the tests weren't as bad as they thought they would be.

During these tests, you may feel dizzy or unsteady. This may make you feel anxious or afraid, which is not uncommon. These feelings generally last just a few minutes and then fade away.

Before your balance exam, tell your audiologist if you're prone to motion sickness. And if, during your tests, you feel uncomfortable or afraid or you want the test to end, speak up. This feedback is helpful for your audiologist, because it offers information that helps isolate the cause of your dizziness. If you have questions before, during or after your tests, bring them up.

After your tests, it's best to have someone drive you home. You may feel tired and a bit unsteady, but these feelings should ease with time.

muscles work together. Electronystag-mography (ENG) is performed using electrodes to collect the information. Videonystagmography (VNG) uses tiny video cameras. These tests are used to study dizziness and vertigo.

Whenever you turn your head, your inner ear tells your brain about this movement. Your brain, in turn, signals your eye muscles in the vestibuloocular reflex. In other words, your eyes move in the opposite direction that you turn your head, which allows you to keep an object in a steady field of vision.

ENG and VNG detect periods of uncontrolled, back-and-forth eye movements (nystagmus). Nystagmus (nis-TAG-mus) may indicate a disorder or injury that's disrupting the vestibuloocular reflex.

For VNG tests, you may be asked to wear special goggles equipped with tiny

infrared cameras. These cameras continually track the movement of your eyes (shown below). If the eye movements are found to occur without any stimuli — for example, without your changing the position of your head — you may be experiencing nystagmus.

For ENG tests, instead of goggles, electrodes are taped at locations around your eyes to record the activity.

To test how well your eye movements respond to signals from your inner ear, you may be asked to stare continuously at a fixed point of light or a spot, follow a point of light with your eyes, follow rotating points of light with your eyes, or lie in different positions while your eye movements are recorded.

You may also have your eye movements tracked with a caloric test. For this test, warm and cool water or air is circulated

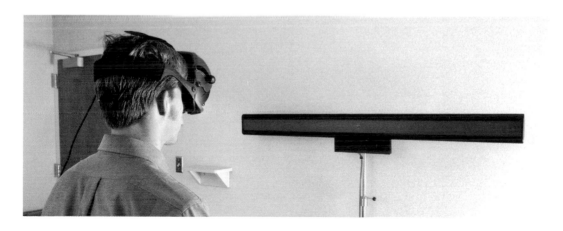

One part of videonystagmography involves following a pinpoint of light with your eyes as it moves across a horizontal electronic bar. This test evaluates how well the brain portions of your balance system control eye movements.

through a soft tube placed in your ear canal. As different temperatures stimulate the inner ear, an audiologist will observe your eye movements.

Video head impulse test

The video head impulse test (vHIT) is a newer form of videonystagmography. It measures how your eyes move in response to short, quick head movements. For this test, you'll wear a lightweight, tightfitting set of goggles and need to keep your neck muscles relaxed.

During the test, your audiologist will ask you to look at a target and move your head back and forth. A computer tracks how well your gaze stays fixed on the target when your head moves. Fast and comfortable, this test is often done with other tests to give a thorough assessment of your inner ear function.

Rotation tests

These tests aren't as common as the other tests you've read about, so not everyone will have them. Because these tests are expensive, not all labs offer them.

Rotation tests tend to be sensitive to inner ear problems. For example, they may show if your balance problems are caused by a medication you're taking. During one form of rotation testing, your audiologist may use electrodes or goggles equipped with infrared cameras to

SHOULD YOU BE CONCERNED ABOUT DIZZINESS?

Generally, any unexplained recurrent or severe spell of dizziness warrants a visit to your doctor. Although it's uncommon for dizziness to signal a serious illness, see your doctor immediately if you experience dizziness or vertigo with any of the following:

- New, different or severe headache
- Blurred vision or double vision
- Hearing loss
- Speech impairment
- Leg or arm weakness
- Loss of consciousness
- Falling or difficulty with walking
- Numbness or tingling
- Chest pain or rapid or slow heart rate

These signs and symptoms may signal the development of a more serious problem.

monitor your eye movements as your body is rotated in different directions and at various speeds. For safety, you're strapped into a chair with a harness and your head is secured against a headrest.

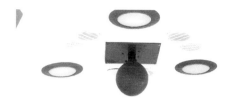

Typically, the testing room is darkened and your audiologist is seated at a computer console just outside the door. A microphone and headset allows you to talk to the audiologist. Often, the computer-controlled chair moves very slowly in a full circle. At faster speeds, it moves back and forth in a very small arc as your eye movements are recorded.

Rather than spinning the chair, the audiologist may have you focus on an object and move your head from side to side or up and down for brief periods. Simplifying the test more, your audiologist may watch your eye movements while he or she manually moves your head or slowly spins you in a swivel chair.

Dix-Hallpike test

The Dix-Hallpike test can determine whether certain movements of your head trigger a form of vertigo known as benign paroxysmal positional vertigo (BPPV). BPPV is characterized by sudden, short bursts of vertigo (see Chapter 15).

You'll start the test sitting on a table. The audiologist may study your eyes directly for the eye movements (nystagmus) characteristic of BPPV. Or you may be asked to wear special goggles equipped with cameras that display the eye movements on a video screen.

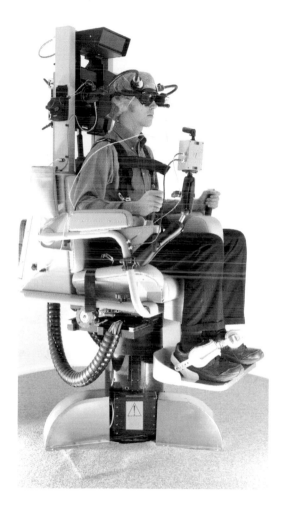

During a rotation test, you may sit in a rotary chair in a darkened room. The audiologist will monitor your eye movements while your body is rotated in the computer-controlled chair in different directions and at different speeds.

Then the following steps will occur:

- The audiologist will move your head to the right or the left at an angle of about 45 degrees.
- You'll move from a sitting position to lying down with your head extended over the edge of the table at the same angle, your head supported by the audiologist.
- The audiologist will observe your eye movement. If nystagmus occurs, it will indicate the location of the problem.

This is done for both ears. If you have BPPV, you'll probably experience vertigo after 2 to 10 seconds of changing position. The sensation may last for 30 seconds to 1 minute. The direction of the nystagmus will tell the audiologist which ear is affected.

Posturography

Posturography tests how well you can integrate sensory information coming from different parts of your balance system: your eyes, the vestibular system in your inner ear, your muscles and joints, and the bottoms of your feet. The exam reveals which elements of the system you've come to rely on most for balance — either on their own or in combination with other elements.

For this test, you'll wear a harness, so it's helpful to wear comfortable clothes. You'll stand on a platform in front of a patterned screen. During the test, a computer will track how well you keep your balance. An audiologist will be close by to help keep you steady if needed.

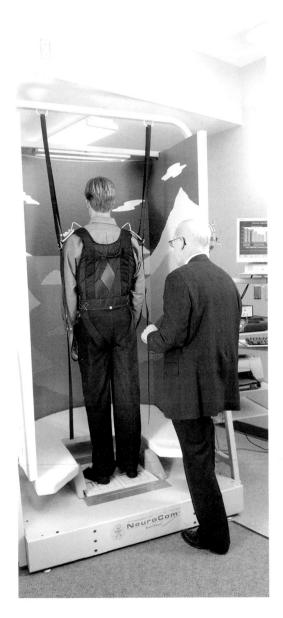

Posturography measures how well you stay balanced when your sensory systems are slightly altered. A platform detects changes in how you distribute your weight as you stand.

Vestibular evoked myogenic potential

A vestibular evoked myogenic potential (VEMP) test collects information about two inner-ear areas that help you balance. To do the test, you lie on your back. The audiologist will put electrodes on the sides of your neck and under your eyes.

In one type of this test, the cervical type (cVEMP), sounds are sent to each ear through small earphones placed in your ears. You'll be asked to lift your head and turn it to the right or left. The electrodes pick up signals from the neck to see if the reflex is working properly.

For the other type of this test, the ocular type (oVEMP), you will either use the same small earphones to hear the sound or the audiologist will place a small device behind your ear to vibrate the bone. The audiologist studies how your eye muscles respond to the stimulation.

Each type of test measures activity in different parts of the balance system and helps diagnose different types of vestibular disorders.

Other tests

Magnetic resonance imaging (MRI) can reveal a variety of conditions, like tumors, that may affect brain structures. Computerized tomography (CT) scans may be used to check for bone fractures or other issues with the skull.

You may also have blood tests to check for an underlying infection. And since blood pressure and circulation can affect dizziness, you may have tests to check the health of your heart and blood vessels.

AFTER A BALANCE EXAM

The tests you have during a balance exam will ideally help your audiologist determine what's causing your dizziness and help set you on a path toward correcting or managing it. In the next chapter, you'll learn about the main types of balance disorders and how they're treated.

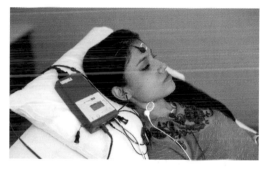

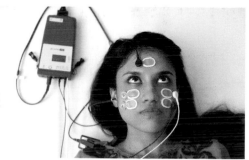

For VEMP testing, you will be asked to contract your neck muscles or look upward to record the response.

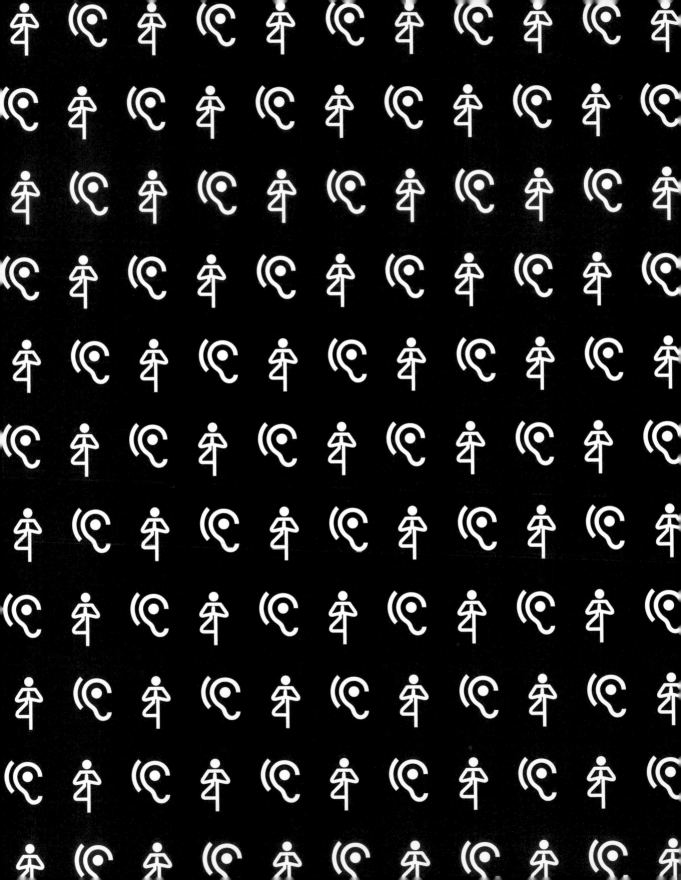

Problems with balance and dizziness

14

Usually, you maintain your sense of balance without thinking about it, based on years of practice and on healthy sensory input. But you've likely experienced brief episodes of dizziness at a point or two in your life. Momentary dizziness is often caused by an abrupt and rapid change in the environment.

You may feel momentarily dizzy when your brain becomes aware of unusual sensory input, like the first time on board a rocking boat. Another example is when you first get off a treadmill — it often takes a few seconds for you to adjust to the fact that your surroundings now move past you when you walk.

Dizziness may also result from conflicting sensory information. For example, if you're sitting in a movie theater watching the shot of a landscape taken through the window of a speeding train, your eyes will signal movement. At the same time, your muscles, nerves and vestibular system tell you that you're stationary. As a result, you may feel dizzy for a moment.

Spinning or sudden movements also cause feelings of dizziness. When you stop moving, the fluid in the inner ears is still in motion for a short time. This is what makes you feel dizzy. When the fluid comes to rest, the dizziness generally goes away.

Dizziness caused by these environmental changes generally isn't serious. But sudden, severe attacks or prolonged episodes of dizziness, faintness, light-headedness or vertigo can be symptoms of an underlying disorder. Sometimes, it's the result of a disruption of the vestibular system.

Following are common non-ear-related causes of balance and dizziness issues.

Low blood pressure

Low blood pressure can make you feel dizzy, lightheaded or faint when you stand up too quickly. The medical term for this is orthostatic hypotension (postural hypotension).

Poor blood circulation

Inadequate blood flow to the brain can cause lightheadedness. Poor blood flow to the inner ear may cause vertigo. Poor circulation may be the result of a heart condition such as blocked arteries or irregular heartbeats (arrhythmia).

Multiple sensory deficits

Lack of input from the eyes, nerves, muscles and joints can make you feel unsteady. Examples include failing vision, nerve damage in the arms and legs (peripheral neuropathy), osteoarthritis, and muscle weakness.

Anxiety disorders

These disorders include panic attacks and a fear of leaving home or being in large, open spaces (agoraphobia). They can make you feel spaced-out or lightheaded.

Even mild forms of situational anxiety can provoke dizziness in some people.

Hyperventilation

Unusually rapid breathing, which often accompanies anxiety disorders, can cause lightheadedness.

Disorders of the central nervous system

These include disorders like Parkinson's disease, multiple sclerosis, tumors and stroke.

Migraines

With or without head pain, migraine events are increasingly recognized as a common cause of dizziness.

Reactions to medications

The action of certain medications can damage the organs of hearing and balance in the inner ear. For this reason, these medications are considered ototoxic (oto- means "ear"). A list of common ototoxic drugs is in Chapter 4. The more medications you take, the more at risk you are of drug-related effects on your hearing and balance systems.

The effects of these medications, which can range from mild to severe, often depend on the doses and the length of time you take them, as well as factors such as kidney and liver function.

Signs and symptoms of ototoxicity include:

- Onset of tinnitus in one or both ears
- Worsening of existing tinnitus
- A feeling that one or both ears are plugged
- Loss of hearing or worsening of existing hearing loss
- Blurred vision when you move your head
- Loss of balance

Make sure that your doctor is aware of any balance or hearing problem whenever you go for a medical visit. Report if you're experiencing balance problems after taking certain medications. This could help you avoid unnecessary exposure to ototoxic drugs.

Imbalance may persist following use of some medications. Vestibular rehabilitation can teach you how to adjust to and cope with the ongoing loss of balance. Learn more in Chapter 16.

The use of alcohol also can cause vertigo and nystagmus, but these symptoms are temporary and usually disappear once the alcohol's effects have subsided. However, the effects of alcohol can last up to 24 hours. Prolonged alcohol abuse can damage parts of the brain and result in permanent issues with imbalance.

VESTIBULAR DISORDERS

If your balance exam suggests that your symptoms are caused by a problem with your balance system (vestibular disorder), you may be diagnosed with an inner ear issue like Ménière's disease, labyrinthitis, vestibular neuritis and acoustic neuroma. You learned about these conditions in Chapter 4. All of these disorders can cause dizziness.

But there are many other conditions that also may lead to dizziness. Here's more on some of the most common vestibular disorders.

Vestibular migraine

The most common cause of vertigo in adults is benign paroxysmal (buh-NINE parok-SIZ-mul) positional vertigo (BPPV). You'll learn about BPPV in Chapter 15.

Vestibular migraine is the second most common cause of vertigo in adults. Migraines have long been associated with dizziness. The dizziness can take any form — spinning, unsteadiness, light-headedness, spontaneous or motion provoked.

This means that the form of dizziness doesn't help determine whether the migraine could be the source of the dizziness. The dizziness that accompanies migraines is episodic, and may not always occur with a headache.

People with vestibular migraine usually have had migraines for years. However, the link between dizziness and migraine hasn't always been well understood.

Today, many people with both headache and dizziness symptoms are diagnosed with vestibular migraine.

While migraine is common in people with vestibular migraine, they also often experience the following signs and symptoms:

- Feeling as if they're moving even though they're not (internal vertigo)
- A false sensation that the room is spinning (external vertigo)
- Sensitivity to sound
- Motion sickness

A vestibular migraine can last just a few minutes or more than 24 hours. The unsteadiness that comes with a vestibular migraine a can last for a day or longer.

Many medications may be used to prevent and treat vestibular migraine. Other strategies include getting adequate sleep, managing stress, staying hydrated, and avoiding diet and lifestyle triggers.

SURGERY FOR VESTIBULAR DISORDERS

Vertigo and other symptoms of vestibular disorders are most often treated with medications or through rehabilitation therapy, but surgery also may be an option. Which option is decided on depends on the frequency and severity of your symptoms, the amount of hearing you've retained, your overall health and your wishes.

Surgery commonly used for vestibular disorders includes:

- Patching a tear in either the oval window or the round window leading from the middle ear to the inner ear (perilymph fistula).
- Placing tissue over a tear at the top of one of the semicircular canals or blocking the canal (superior semicircular canal dehiscence).
- Draining excess fluid (endolymph) from the endolymphatic sac that's located near the mastoid bone behind your ear. This is called endolymphatic decompression surgery.
- Cutting the vestibular nerve (vestibular nerve section) at a location before it joins with the auditory nerve. This procedure can potentially eliminate vertigo while preserving your hearing. It may be a reasonable option for a younger person with severe symptoms of Ménière's disease and no other significant medical problems.
- Destroying the inner ear (labyrinthectomy). This is a relatively simple operation with fewer risks than in vestibular nerve section. Because the procedure destroys the labyrinth, it's usually reserved for those who have no usable hearing in the affected ear. After surgery, the brain gradually adjusts, compensating for the loss of the balance mechanism in one ear by relying on the functioning mechanism of the other ear. Vestibular and balance therapy can help hasten this compensation process.

Persistent postural-perceptual dizziness

Another cause of dizziness is persistent postural-perceptual dizziness (PPPD), a condition commonly associated with vestibular disorders, migraines, anxiety, panic attacks and a nervous system disorder called dysautonomia. Persistent dizziness typically occurs with movement and is made worse by environments with a lot of movement, like being in crowds or in a grocery store, movie theater or airport. Tasks that require hand-eye coordination may be difficult. This condition used to be known as chronic subjective dizziness syndrome (CSD).

PPPD is a conditioned response that develops out of the anxiety that may result when dizziness occurs from another cause. Medications used to treat anxiety or depression may help control the condition, as can vestibular and balance therapy.

Third window disorders

A third window disorder happens when there is a defect in the bony structure of the inner ear. These disorders usually cause sound- or pressure-induced vertigo. There are several conditions that are classified as third window disorders, including perilymph fistula and superior semicircular canal dehiscence.

Perilymph fistula

A perilymph fistula is a tear or other defect that allows fluid (perilymph) from the inner ear to leak into the air-filled middle ear.

The condition is often caused by head trauma but can also be caused by rapid changes in atmospheric pressure, experienced during activities like scuba diving or airplane maneuvers. It may also occur due to extreme exertion, like heavy lifting or childbirth.

The condition is controversial because the holes or defects in the membrane are so small and exceedingly difficult to detect — which can often make diagnosis difficult.

Signs and symptoms of perilymph fistula may include vertigo, imbalance, nausea and vomiting. A fistula may also lead to tinnitus and hearing loss.

Bed rest and avoiding sudden movements often allow the rupture to heal on its own. If this doesn't work, surgery may be performed to repair the tiny opening.

Superior semicircular canal dehiscence

Superior semicircular canal dehiscence (SSCD) is a type of fistula involving an unusual opening in the inner ear. But with SSCD, the opening is at the top of one of the semicircular canals of the vestibular labyrinth, where there's a lack of bone covering the canal.

The primary symptom associated with SSCD is dizziness when straining — for example, when lifting something heavy — or when hearing loud noises such as

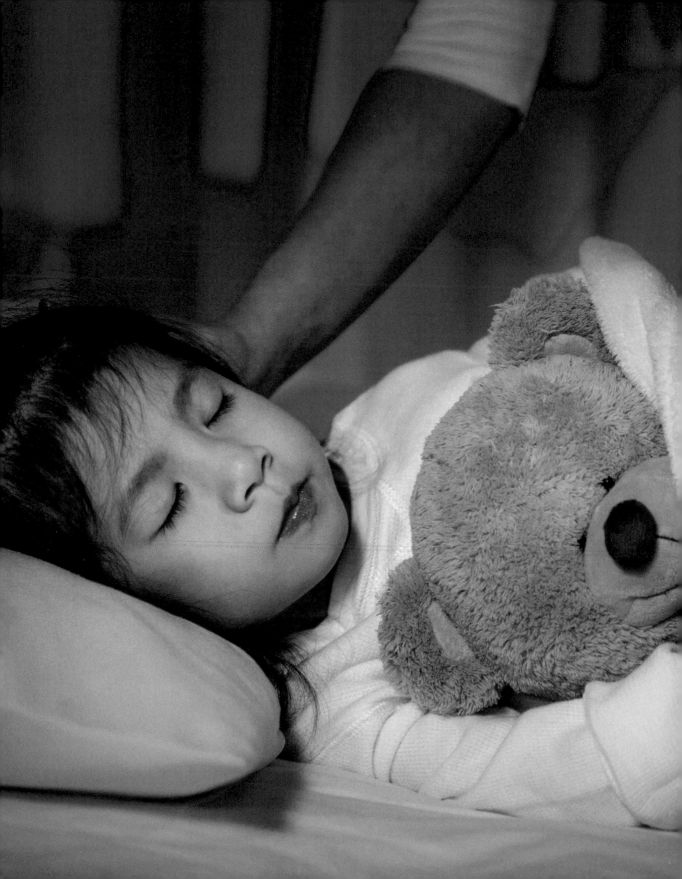

dog barks. Some people even hear internal body sounds like their heartbeats or eyes moving. The condition may involve a specific type of hearing loss.

While not easy to diagnose, SSCD is far less controversial than is an oval or round window fistula. That's because the opening on the semicircular canal can be detected with a CT scan or from certain audiological tests. Surgery can often repair the defect, relieving dizziness and returning hearing to typical levels.

DIZZINESS IN CHILDREN

Children of all ages can have problems with dizziness and balance. While they're not as common as in adults, children may be affected by many of the same disorders. The most common disorder in children is migraine-related dizziness. In younger children, an ear infection also is a common cause of dizziness.

The child's description of his or her dizziness, along with any observations that can be provided by parents or other caregivers are key parts of an evaluation. All of the tests used to evaluate dizziness in adults can be used for children, with modifications — such as the child sitting on his or her parent's lap during the rotary chair test — if necessary. A hearing evaluation also will be completed.

Children are treated for dizziness issues much in the same way adults are. For migraine issues, medications can be used when needed, but rest in a dark, quiet room also is helpful.

BALANCE AND DIZZINESS ARE TREATABLE

Most of the time, vestibular problems aren't life-threatening, and your doctor can prescribe ways to manage the condition. The key is to work together with your health care team to find the best blend of therapies to address your symptoms. In the next section, you'll learn about strategies to manage balance issues and cope with chronic dizziness on a daily basis.

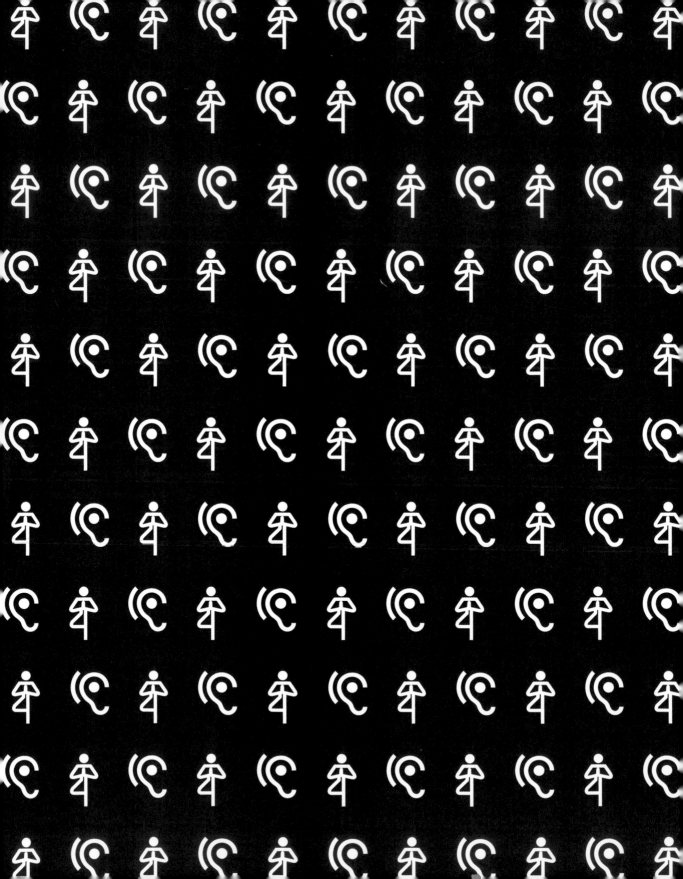

15

BPPV

Teresa was helping her friend pack for a move. At one point, Teresa was reaching up into a cupboard, pulling down glasses one by one, wrapping them and placing them in a box. "The next morning," Teresa says, "I woke up swirling and nauseated. The nausea was relieved only if I laid on one side."

Teresa then had a similar experience when she helped another friend hang pictures on a wall. She was constantly looking up and down. "Once again," Teresa says, "the next morning I had the swirling sensation and nausea."

These symptoms continue to this day anytime Teresa bends her head. She also started to have balance problems. Teresa's doctor diagnosed her with benign paroxysmal (par-ok-SIZ-mul) positional vertigo (BPPV). BPPV is the most common cause of vertigo that's linked to a problem with the balance system. Of all the people who see a doctor for dizziness, nearly half are diagnosed with BPPV.

In this chapter, you'll get an up-close look at this condition and how to manage it.

WHAT IS BPPV?

The inner ear houses an intricate system that helps with balance. Earlier in this book, you learned that the balance system of the inner ear consists of three loop-shaped tubes (semicircular canals). These tubes contain fluid that monitors the rotation of the head. These tubes attach to a sac-like structure called the utricle.

Within the utricle are tiny crystals called otoconia. These tiny crystals are attached to sensors that help you detect gravity and straight-line motion. These sensors, in turn, send messages through the vestibular nerve to the brain. This process helps you maintain your balance.

With BPPV, the tiny crystals that help you stay balanced get dislodged. They move from the part of the inner ear where they usually do their job to another part of the inner ear. When these tiny crystals move out of place, you may feel as if you're spinning or moving. You may also lose your balance, feel unsteady, become nauseated or vomit.

An episode of BPPV may be triggered by a change in head position. This can occur when you get in or out of bed, turn over in bed, tilt your head to look up, look over your shoulder, or sit up. This sensation is sudden, brief and often severe. An episode may last seconds to minutes.

Nearly a third of people who have one BPPV episode will have another one. This disorder is twice as common in women as it is in men. BPPV often shows up in a person's late 40s or early 50s. Episodes happen more often with age.

About half the people with BPPV also have balance issues. They're more likely to have trouble walking, using stairs or walking on unstable surfaces.

While BPPV is the most common cause of vertigo in adults, children can have it, too. It's usually associated with minor trauma, hormonal changes or migraines.

RISK FACTORS

Often, there's no known cause for BPPV. When there is a known cause, BPPV is often associated with a minor to severe blow to the head.

Less common causes of BPPV include disorders that damage your inner ear. Rarely, damage that occurs during ear surgery or long periods positioned on your back can cause BPPV, for example, when sitting in a dentist chair or when recovering from an illness.

Some research shows that people with BPPV between ages 18 and 39 have several risk factors in common. These include doing yoga or running on paved surfaces, working underneath cars, and reaching up high for things. Intense aerobic activity, jogging, running on a treadmill and swimming also have been linked to cases of BPPV in this age group.

In people older than age 40 with BPPV, head trauma and other ear disorders, like vestibular neuritis or labyrinthitis, are common.

Although BPPV is uncomfortable, it rarely causes complications. But the dizziness of BPPV can make you unsteady, which may put you at greater risk of falling.

TESTS YOU MAY HAVE

At your appointment with your doctor, you may be asked these questions:
• What are your symptoms?

- When did you first notice the symptoms you're experiencing?
- Do your symptoms come and go? How often?
- How long do your symptoms last?
- Does anything in particular seem to trigger your symptoms, such as certain types of movement or activity?
- Do your symptoms include vision problems?
- Do your symptoms include nausea or vomiting?
- Do your symptoms include headache?
- Have you lost any hearing?
- Are you being treated for any other medical conditions?

If your doctor thinks your symptoms may be caused by BPPV, you'll likely have a series of tests, starting with basic hearing and balance exams.

Then, you'll likely have tests that help show whether:
- Your signs and symptoms of dizziness are prompted by eye or head movements and then decrease in less than one minute
- Dizziness is linked to specific eye movements that occur when you lie on your back with your head turned to one side and tipped slightly over the edge of the examination bed
- Your eyes move from side to side on their own
- You have trouble controlling your eye movements

If these tests don't reveal the cause of your signs and symptoms, other tests may be needed, including tests to detect eye movement or create images of your head.

Electronystagmography (ENG) or videonystagmography (VNG)

These tests detect irregular eye movement. ENG uses electrodes and VNG uses small cameras. Either test can help determine whether dizziness is due to inner ear disease. These tests work by measuring involuntary eye movements while your head is placed in different positions or your balance organs are stimulated with water or air.

Magnetic resonance imaging (MRI)

This test uses a magnetic field and radio waves to create cross-sectional images of your head and body. Your doctor can use these images to identify and diagnose a range of conditions. MRI may be performed to rule out other possible causes of vertigo.

Your primary doctor can often diagnose and treat BPPV, but you may need to see an ear, nose and throat specialist (ENT), a physical therapist, or an audiologist.

HOW BPPV IS TREATED

BPPV may go away on its own within a few weeks or months. But, to relieve symptoms sooner, you may have treatment in your doctor's office or with an audiologist or physical therapist.

The goal of BPPV treatment is to direct the tiny crystals in the inner ear that help you stay balanced to the part of the inner ear where they need to be. This is done

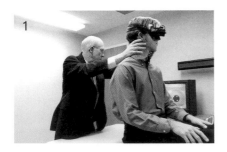

To help relieve BPPV, your audiologist may help you perform a series of maneuvers known as the canalith repositioning procedure. Each step is held for about 30 to 60 seconds. This example is for BPPV on the left side.

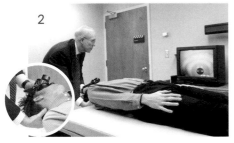

1. Start in a seated position with your head turned at a 45-degree angle to the left.

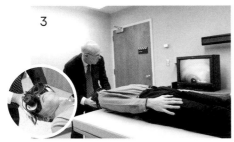

2. Move to a reclining position while keeping your head at the same angle. The audiologist supports your head as it extends over the edge of the table.

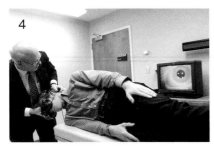

3. Still reclined, turn your head to the right.

4. Roll over on your side. Your head is angled slightly as you look down at the floor.

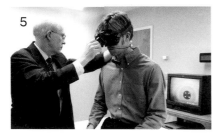

5. Return carefully to a sitting position with your chin tilted down.

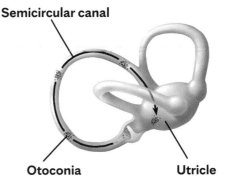

Semicircular canal

Otoconia

Utricle

As you work through the procedure, the loose otoconia return to the area of the utricle.

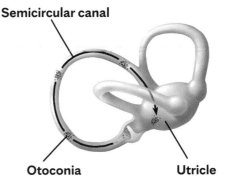

with a series of exercises that involve maneuvering your head. While there are medications that can be used for dizziness, they're not as effective as repositioning procedures.

BPPV is typically treated with a series of movements known as the canalith repositioning procedure.

Canalith repositioning procedure

The canalith repositioning procedure, also known as Epley's maneuver, involves holding four positions for about 30 seconds each, or as long as you have symptoms in a position. It's typical to stay in each position an extra 30 seconds after symptoms have stopped. The doctor watches for irregular eye movements during the procedure. The procedure may be repeated three or more times within a one session. One or two treatments resolve symptoms for most people.

Doctors often teach people how to do these exercises at home. Then, when symptoms arise, people can do the exercises twice each day, once in the morning and again in the afternoon. Some people may need to continue doing the exercises twice a day until three days go by with no symptoms. Ask your doctor for specific instructions.

When you do these exercises at home, keep your head in an upright position for

EVERYDAY TIPS FOR DIZZINESS FROM BPPV

If your dizziness is caused by BPPV, these suggestions may help.

- If your dizziness is caused by BPPV, be aware of the possibility of losing your balance. Loss of balance can lead to falling and serious injury.
- Sit or lie down right away when you feel dizzy.
- When sleeping, don't lie on the side of your affected ear.
- Get out of bed slowly and sit on the edge of the bed for a minute.
- Avoid movements that bring on symptoms, like bending down or looking up.
- Avoid extending your head backward, such as when getting something from an upper cabinet.
- Be careful when getting up from lying back at the dentist's office, beauty salon or barbershop, or during activities like yoga or massage.
- When you're in bed, place pillows under your head to avoid lying completely flat.
- Use nightlights to help you see in the dark.
- Use a cane for stability.

20 minutes afterward. You can look right or left and move around, but don't tilt your head up or down during that time.

These exercises aren't a cure for BPPV, but they can help most people manage its symptoms. If you try these exercises and they don't help, you may need more treatment sessions with your doctor, audiologist or physical therapist.

Rarely, the canalith repositioning procedure may not work, and your doctor may recommend surgery. In this surgery, a bone plug is used to block the portion of your inner ear that's causing dizziness. The plug prevents the affected semicircular canal in your ear from being able to respond to particle movements or head movements in general.

Other home exercises

In addition to the canalith repositioning procedure, there are other exercises you can do at home when you have symptoms of BPPV. For most people, symptoms of vertigo go away after doing these exercises for a few days.

SUE'S STORY: 'A RELIEF TO FINALLY HAVE A DIAGNOSIS'

Sue's bouts of dizziness started in her teens. Sometimes she had to keep her head level and not look down for weeks at a time. None of this was a surprise, considering her dad had dizziness spells, too, and many generations of her family were treated for similar issues.

But later on in life, Sue's episodes worsened. They became more frequent and more violent, and they lasted for five days or more. Her doctor ordered several tests, including a brain scan to rule out a tumor. From there, Sue's doctor referred her to a dizziness and balance clinic. After many more tests, Sue was diagnosed with BPPV. About five days after being treated with the canalith repositioning procedure, Sue started to feel better.

Just having an answer was helpful for Sue. Even better, she learned how to do the canalith repositioning procedure at home.

"It was a relief to finally have a diagnosis, and to know after all those years, that there was something I could do to help," Sue says.

Now, at the first sign of dizziness, she does these exercises for three to five days. "Usually, this prevents a full-blown attack," Sue says. "I feel like I can keep BPPV managed pretty well."

Gufoni maneuver

Do this exercise once a day until you go three days without any BPPV symptoms. Take these steps:
- Sit on the edge of a bed.
- Lie straight on your side with a small pillow under your head. Stay in this position for 30 seconds.
- Turn your face down toward the pillow for 30 seconds. Don't turn your body.
- Keep your head turned as you sit back up slowly.
- Turn your head straight with your chin down slightly.
- Sit for one minute before you get up.

Passive nighttime positioning

This exercise is also called forced-prolonged positioning. Do this exercise once a day until you go three days without any BPPV symptoms.

First, lie on one side for 30 to 60 seconds. Then, roll onto your other side. Stay on this side all night. If you get up in the night, lie back on one side for 30 to 60 seconds. Then roll to your other side for the rest of the night.

A MANAGEABLE CONDITION

BPPV is a balance disorder that's likely to recur from time to time, especially in those whose condition is related to trauma. It's common, especially with age. While the impact of this condition can range from mild to severe, with the right plan in place, you can manage the symptoms of this condition.

Living well with balance issues and dizziness

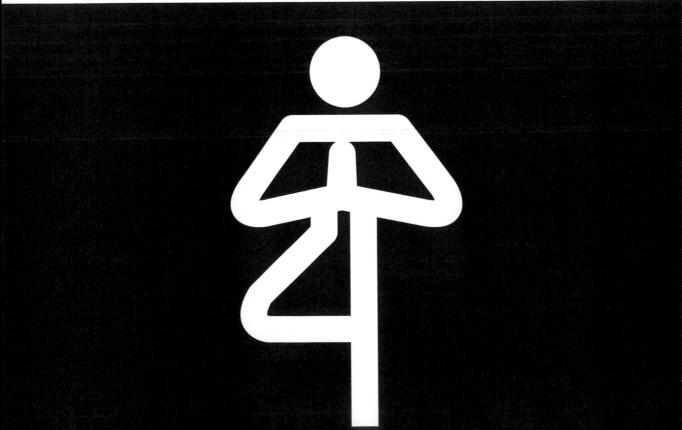

PART 6

Managing balance issues

Balance problems are common. As people age, they tend to be less active and their bodies gradually lose the fine balance skills of their youth.

Are problems with balance taking a toll on you physically, mentally or emotionally? If you said yes, you're not alone.

If you're afraid of falling, you may avoid situations that increase your risk, preferring to keep to yourself and stay home. You may forgo the activities of life that bring you meaning and joy. This is likely at least part of the reason why as many as half of the people with vestibular disorders develop anxiety, depression or panic disorders.

Balance disorders have physical effects, as well. If you worry about falling, you

may move less — or not at all. Moving less makes it more likely that you'll lose muscle tone, muscle strength and the balance skills you do have. Your posture may change over time, altering the way you move and making balance difficult.

Balance and dizziness issues can be part of a vicious cycle. But with the right daily choices and types and amounts of activity, you can sidestep their negative mental, emotional and physical effects. In this chapter, you'll learn what steps to take.

START AT HOME

The choices you make at home can either make falls more likely or less likely. As you chart your course toward better balance, start by looking at your home environment. The choices you make can help you feel more comfortable.

Remove home hazards

Take a look around. Your living room, kitchen, bedroom, bathroom, hallways and stairways may be filled with hazards.

You may reduce home hazards by:
- Removing boxes, newspapers, electrical cords and phone cords from walkways
- Moving coffee tables, magazine racks and plant stands from high-traffic areas
- Securing loose rugs with double-faced tape, tacks or a slip-resistant backing
- Storing clothing, dishes, food and other necessities within easy reach
- Immediately cleaning up spilled liquids, grease or food
- Using nonskid floor wax
- Using nonslip mats in the bathtub or shower

If needed, ask your health care team about getting an occupational therapist's tips for reducing your fall risk at home.

Light up your living space

Some tripping hazards are hard to see. Keeping your home brightly lit can help.

Consider these adjustments:
- Place night lights in your bedroom, bathroom and hallways.
- Place a lamp within reach of your bed for middle-of-the-night needs.
- Store flashlights in easy-to-find places in case of power outages.

- Turn on lights before using the stairs.
- Make clear paths to light switches that aren't near room entrances.
- Trade traditional switches for glow-in-the-dark or illuminated switches.
- Consider installing motion sensor lighting that automatically turns on and off when you enter and leave the area. You can even find lightbulbs that serve this purpose for light fixtures you already have.

Use assistive devices

If your doctor recommends using a cane or walker, ask whether a physical therapist can help you choose the best device for you and teach you how to use it.

Other assistive devices can help, too. For example:
- Handrails for both sides of stairways
- Nonslip treads for bare-wood steps
- A raised toilet seat or one with armrests
- Grab bars for the shower or tub
- A sturdy plastic seat for the shower or tub — plus a hand-held shower nozzle
- A phone with preprogrammed speed dial for emergency contacts to have next to your bed

Wear sensible shoes

Consider changing your footwear as part of your fall-prevention plan. High heels, floppy slippers or sandals, and shoes with slick soles can make it more likely that you'll slip, stumble and fall. So can walking in your stocking feet.

Make sure your shoes are firmly attached to your feet, keeping your toes and heels in place. This provides a direct line of communication between your feet and your brain. Your brain tells the muscles in your feet what adjustments they need to make to keep you steady.

TALK TO YOUR HEALTH CARE TEAM

Several areas of fall risk are best assessed by your health care team. At your next appointment, discuss your concerns and areas of your life that may be helping or hurting your balance.

Be prepared to discuss these topics.

Medications

Make a list of all the prescription and over-the-counter medications and supplements you take, or bring them with you to the appointment. Your health care team can review your medications for side effects and interactions that may increase your risk of falling.

If you take several medications and supplements, consider using a pill dispenser. This helps ensure that you're taking medications as prescribed, rather than taking too little or too much.

Fall history

Have you fallen before? If you've landed on the ground or a lower surface unexpectedly, this counts as a fall — even if your dog tripped you, or you got tangled up in bedsheets.

It's important to report every instance of a fall. People who've fallen once are more likely to fall again. Write down all the details, including when, where and how you fell. The details you provide can help your health care team identify specific fall-prevention strategies.

Health conditions and overall health

Talk about any health conditions you have and discuss how comfortable you are when you walk. Posture and body alignment also are important. When you're in proper alignment while sitting, standing and walking, your joints and muscles will likely work more efficiently, and your balance muscles won't have to work so hard to keep you on your feet. Your health care team may test your muscle strength, balance and walking style (gait).

If you have Parkinson's disease, multiple sclerosis or another chronic neurological condition that alters your balance, working with a physical therapist on a home exercise program may help. Your exercise program can be reevaluated every year or as your condition changes.

When you meet with your health care team, ask how often you should have eye exams. If you need corrective lenses, consider having two pairs of glasses if you have trouble seeing far away and close up. Multifocal lenses like progressive lenses and bifocals can make a fall more likely, especially on uneven ground, when stepping onto or off of curbs, or when using stairs. Consider surgery if you have cataracts.

Pain is another important part of overall health. Pain makes it harder to respond to balance challenges.

Do you have foot or ankle pain? Leg or back pain? Talk with your health care team about specialists who may be able to help. Your health care team can also help you come up with a plan to keep pain under control.

Lifestyle

Your daily habits are critical to good balance. When you meet with your health care team, be prepared to answer these questions.

Are you a risk taker?

Do you climb a ladder that you shouldn't to change a lightbulb, trim a tree or take a look at a leak in your roof? If you're doing things that others think you shouldn't because they're unsafe, think again before making that next choice. A fall from a height can change your life. Is it worth the risk?

Are you physically active?

Physical activity can go a long way toward fall prevention. If your health care team feels it's safe, consider activities like walking, water workouts, dancing or tai chi. These activities improve strength, balance, coordination and flexibility. If you're not comfortable with exercise, ask your health care team about working with a physical therapist to create a physical activity plan that meets your needs.

Are you avoiding physical activity because you're afraid that you'll fall? Share your concerns with your health care team. As you learned at the beginning of this chapter, not getting enough physical activity is likely to weaken your muscles and make balance issues worse. Your health care team may be able to offer exercise programs for your situation or refer you to a physical therapist.

Are you socially active?

According to research, people who connect with family and friends are less likely to fall. Research also suggests that those who are married or live with someone are more likely to have a fall-prevention plan.

Do you drink alcohol?

Alcohol decreases your reaction time. It may also impair your ability to adjust quickly when your balance is challenged.

Are you anxious, depressed or not getting enough sleep?

All of these conditions can make you less aware of your surroundings. As a result, you may be more likely to fall. Talk with your health care team about ways to improve your health in these areas. Managing anxiety and depression and getting good sleep all help with balance.

VESTIBULAR REHABILITATION

Dizziness and vertigo frequently go away on their own. But sometimes they persist. If you experience dizziness, vertigo or other signs and symptoms of a vestibular disorder that disrupt your life for several weeks or more, your doctor may refer you to a physical therapist for vestibular rehabilitation.

Vestibular rehabilitation is an effective therapeutic program that uses physical exercise and head and body movements to decrease your symptoms and help you regain your sense of balance. Vestibular rehabilitation is frequently recommended after inner ear surgery, but it's often used on its own, as well. These programs are usually led by a physical therapist or an occupational therapist. They're useful for anyone, at any age.

Adapting to change

Vestibular rehabilitation helps you stay active and learn to maintain your everyday routine despite balance concerns. This form of therapy helps the balance-related parts of your brain, central nervous system and musculoskeletal system adapt to the changes you're experiencing. You may hear adaptation referred to as compensation.

When your vestibular system is damaged, your brain receives conflicting messages about movement and your body's position in space. This is what causes dizziness. You may try to avoid rapid movements at first to avoid symptoms of dizziness.

But remaining relatively inactive for long periods of time doesn't stimulate your brain to do what it needs to do — change and adapt. Inactivity also decreases your muscle strength and flexibility.

Adaptation often occurs naturally with experience, as you move around and carry out daily activities. In order for your brain to adapt, it needs to continue receiving signals from the balance organs — even if the signals aren't typical. In time, the brain usually resets by using other sources of sensory input.

For example, if your inner ear on the left side stops working, your balance system may rely more on the organs in your right ear gradually over time. When this compensation is complete, you'll rarely notice the dizziness.

You may wonder about taking anti-vertigo medications for balance and dizziness issues in place of vestibular rehabilitation. While these medications are important for relieving acute spells of dizziness, long-term therapeutic use of these drugs is discouraged. That's because they're mostly sedative in nature, and in the long run, they may delay the brain's ability to compensate.

At times, the signs and symptoms of a balance disorder become chronic. This increases the risk of falls and injuries. In older adults, falls are a major cause of disability and death.

This highlights another value of vestibular rehabilitation: It can be an important way to prevent falls.

Balance disorders affect people physically and emotionally, making it essential to find treatments that address both aspects. The following integrative approaches have been used alongside traditional treatments to manage chronic dizziness and the mental health issues that can arise from both.

Cognitive behavioral therapy

In recent years, there has been an increased focus on using cognitive approaches to treat dizziness. Cognitive behavioral therapy is used to treat various conditions, including anxiety and depression, which commonly occur alongside balance issues. This therapy aims to change the way people think about their health problems and give people the tools to better respond to their problems.

Cognitive behavioral therapy can help replace negative thoughts about balance disorders. For example, *I'll never be able to get this dizziness under control!* can be replaced with more-realistic and positive thoughts, such as *I now know what my triggers are, and I'm going to learn how to avoid them.* The therapy also teaches ways to cope with stressful life situations, which can worsen these health problems.

Research suggests that cognitive behavioral therapy, combined with vestibular rehabilitation, reduces dizziness, improves walking, and results in less anxiety and depression in people with persistent dizziness. Cognitive behavioral therapy can help people identify dizziness triggers, which may allow them to avoid anxiety.

Mindfulness

Stress is a known trigger for dizziness. "Moving meditation" exercises such as yoga, tai chi and Pilates may help improve balance and help with stress management through controlled breathing, relaxation and guided imagery. Yoga, for example, can help quiet the mind and reduce anxiety. Specific yoga poses for balance include the warrior, tree and triangle poses.

People with balance issues should take precautions while practicing these exercises, ensuring that balancing aids — such as a chair or wall — are nearby.

Biofeedback

Biofeedback helps people adapt to a balance disorder. Movement follows a cycle: An action is started and performed, and any movement errors are detected. A biofeedback device gathers this information about the body, offering a snapshot of how it reacts to a specific movement. Using this information, a person with balance issues can make adjustments to help improve balance.

Various devices offer biofeedback for balance issues. One type has plates that a person stands on, measuring how much the person sways while standing still. Another provides feedback on how balance issues may be affecting a person as he or she walks.

Coaching

Patient education is key part of managing all aspects of balance dysfunction. As part of a comprehensive treatment plan, health care providers work to inform patients about their conditions, including abilities, limitations, and whether this may be a short-term or long-term problem. They provide coaching on how to perform balancing-improvement tasks and how to adapt or modify movements should the task or situation change.

Providers also focus on the patient's environment — such as the home or work environment — and what challenges and safety issues may exist in these places for someone who has chronic dizziness. An evaluation to look at potential home hazards, such as poor lighting and slippery floor surfaces, may be recommended. Modifications such as adding brighter lighting, installing handrails, placing phones near floor level (in case of a fall), and selecting footwear that's less of a trip or slip hazard may be discussed.

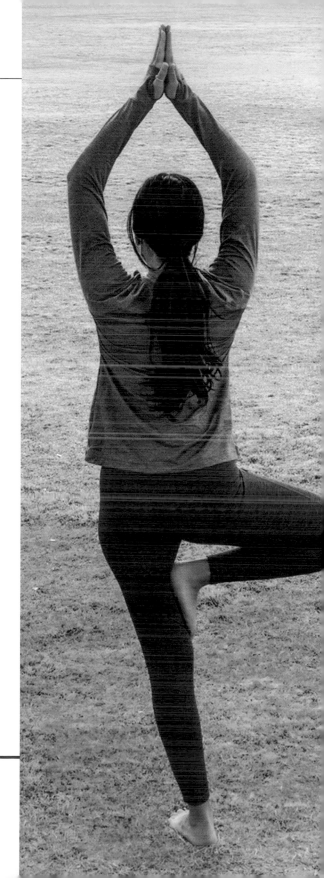

What's in a program?

A vestibular rehabilitation program generally starts with a thorough assessment of your signs and symptoms and underlying conditions. This allows a physical therapist to design an exercise program customized to your needs.

The assessment typically includes:
- An evaluation of your strength, coordination and flexibility skills.
- Balance and gait assessments that are compared with those of others in your age group. These assessments also test how well your balance organs work together.
- Questions about how frequent and severe your symptoms are, when and where they occur, and what factors might make them worse.
- A test to rate your level of dizziness as you change in and out of various positions.
- An evaluation of how well you control your eye movement while your head is in motion.
- A list of activities you're avoiding and which ones you'd like to do.

With a better understanding of your situation, your therapist can help you set goals, like improving your eye movement control and increasing your activity levels. Your therapist can also advise you on how to reach these goals.

Typically, your therapist will recommend a number of exercises to do at home, in between your visits. Your therapist will likely encourage you to move your head, eyes and body in a safe manner even though these motions may increase your dizziness or challenge your balance.

For example, you may be asked to watch a target at arm's length and move your head quickly to the right and left while keeping the target in focus. This activity can be repeated several times a day. Other simple exercises may include focusing on a visual target 5 to 10 feet away while moving from a sitting position to a standing position and back again with your eyes open. You may then be asked to repeat the procedure with your eyes closed.

At first these exercises may make you dizzy, so you'll start out doing only a few at a time. Your brain will likely get used to these movements, finding ways to compensate for your vestibular injury. You'll gradually increase how long and intensely you perform these exercises. Dizziness usually fades away.

You may also be given exercises to increase your strength and coordination — in other words, improve your balance control. This might include a daily walking program. The best general suggestion is to get back into your normal, active daily routine as quickly as you can. This means performing activities that require you to move your body, head and eyes. Loading and unloading the dishwasher is a practical example.

STAYING ACTIVE

After you finish a therapy program, it's important to stay physically active. Many

SIT-TO-STAND TEST

Many factors can make it more or less likely that you'll fall. One important factor is the strength in your legs. If you're not sure how strong your legs are, take this 30-second sit-to-stand test.

Here's how to do it:
- Use a chair with a standard height, about 17 inches from the floor.
- Sit close to the front of the chair.
- Stand all the way up and sit down as many times as you can in 30 seconds.

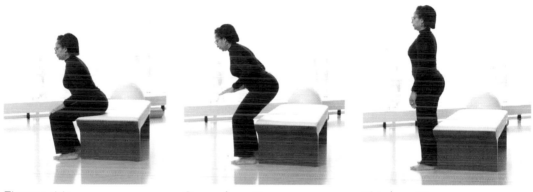

First position   Second position   Third position

The more repetitions you can do, the lower your risk is of falling. In general, physical therapists say that those who can't do at least eight repetitions have a higher risk of falling. How many repetitions did you do?

Use this chart to compare your results against others in your age range.

Ages	60-64	65-69	70-74	75-79	80-84	85-89	90-94
Women	12-17	11-16	10-15	10-15	9-14	8-13	4-11
Men	14-19	12-18	12-17	11-17	10-15	8-14	7-12

Source: Centers for Disease Control and Prevention

If it's hard to stand up from standard-height chair, start your practice with a higher bed or stool. Or try placing a pillow on the seat of the chair. As you practice, do each repetition as slowly as possible. The longer you take for each repetition, the more muscle strength you'll build in your legs.

people choose tai chi to maintain leg strength and balance, but the most critical point is to choose activities that keep you moving and help you keep your balance system in good working order. Talk to your health care team about which exercises are best for you.

If your body goes through a period of inactivity, such as during a bout with the flu or after minor surgery, your brain may forget some of its compensation methods. To correct this, you'll need to retrain your balance system.

You can do this by regularly performing the exercises you learned until the dizziness go away. Generally, the signs and symptoms will recede more quickly the second time around.

A SIMPLE BALANCE TEST

Simple exercises can improve your balance. The key to achieving better balance is to find exercises and activities that are safe but challenging. The more you consistently challenge your brain and body, the more your balance abilities are likely to improve.

Start by taking the test on the next page. Find a safe area where you have support if you need it. You might use a corner where two walls meet or stand close to a bed or next to a countertop.

How did it go? Did you make it to the last exercise? If so, how long did you stand on one foot? Compare your results against others in your age group by using the table to the right.

If you feel confident doing each of these exercises, try them again. This time, stand on the other foot or close your eyes while doing the exercises. Make sure you have support nearby if you need it.

Age	Eyes open	Eyes closed
18-39	43	9.4
40-49	40	7.3
50-59	37	4.8
60-69	27	2.8
70-79	15	2.0
80-99	6.2	1.3

Source: Springer BA, et al. Normative values for the unipedal stance test with eyes open and closed. Journal of Geriatric Physical Therapy. 2007; doi:10.1519/00139143-200704000-00003.

Were some of the standing balance exercises hard for you? For example, did you sway a little during an exercise? Was there a position you couldn't quite hold for 10 seconds without support? The answers to these questions will tell you which exercises, featured on the following pages, to do next.

MAKE BALANCE A DAILY HABIT

You can do balance exercises anywhere, anytime. Even simple exercises, when you do them often, can help you boost your balance.

Try standing in a balance-challenging position while you're brushing your teeth or waiting in line at the grocery store. Walk on your tiptoes. Exercise classes are another option. Whether they're in person at your local community center or online, tai chi and dancing are examples of the types of classes that can help you improve your balance in a fun and engaging way.

Choose activities that you can do safely — but that challenge you. If you need more help with your balance, ask your doctor about trying physical therapy.

	Stand with your feet side by side.	Can you hold this position without stepping or touching a wall for 10 seconds? Hold your arms out to the side (easier) or crossed over your chest (harder). If you feel confident while performing this exercise for 10 seconds, proceed to the next position.	**Time:** _____ seconds
	Place the instep of one foot so that it's touching the big toe of the other foot.	Can you hold this position for 10 seconds without touching a wall or taking a step? If so, proceed to the next exercise.	**Time:** _____ seconds
	Tandem stand: Place one foot in front of the other, heel touching toe.	Try holding this stance for 10 seconds without stepping or touching. If you can't, you have a higher risk of falling.	**Time:** _____ seconds
	Stand on one foot.	When you try this exercise, don't let your legs touch.	**Time:** _____ seconds

Source: Centers for Disease Control and Prevention

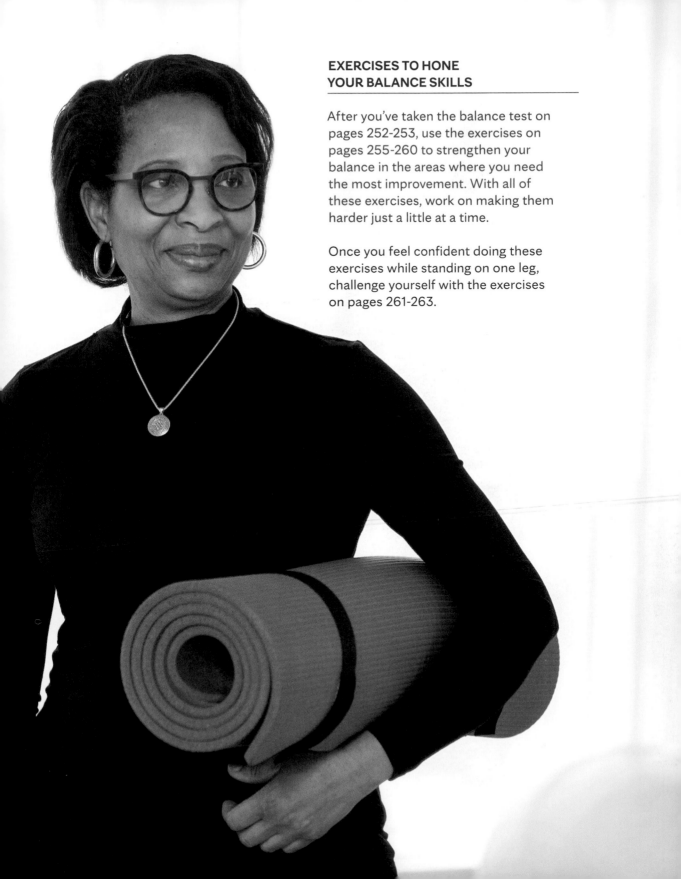

EXERCISES TO HONE YOUR BALANCE SKILLS

After you've taken the balance test on pages 252-253, use the exercises on pages 255-260 to strengthen your balance in the areas where you need the most improvement. With all of these exercises, work on making them harder just a little at a time.

Once you feel confident doing these exercises while standing on one leg, challenge yourself with the exercises on pages 261-263.

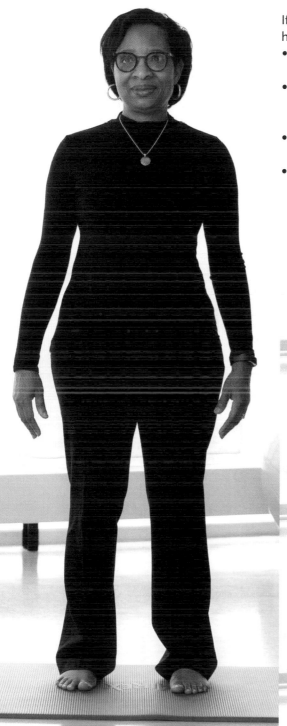

If standing with your feet side by side was hard for you:

- Stand with your feet at a comfortable distance apart.
- Try shifting your weight without lifting your feet off the ground from the right to the left side.
- Stand with one foot forward as if you are taking a step.
- Shift your weight to the forward foot and then to the back foot without lifting your feet off the ground.

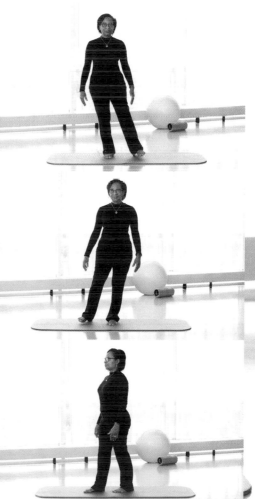

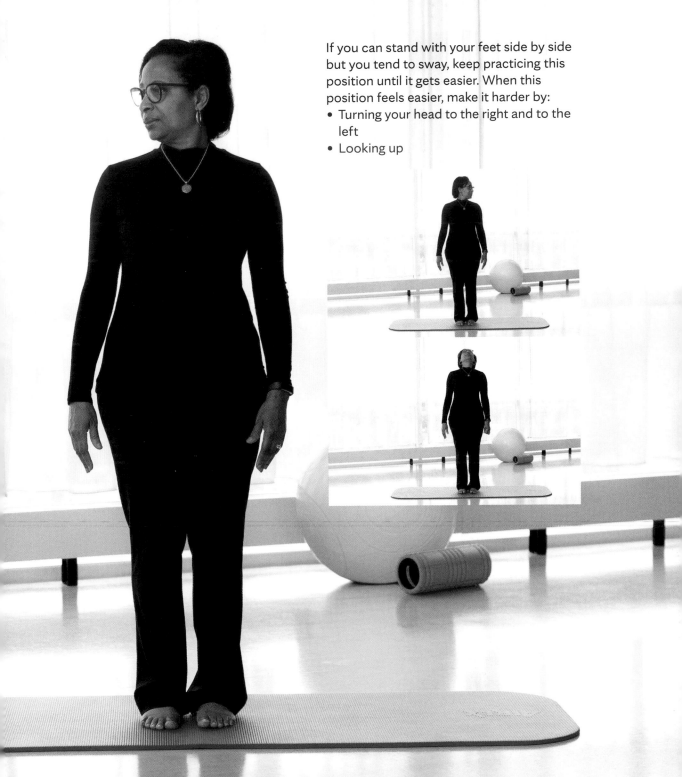

If you can stand with your feet side by side but you tend to sway, keep practicing this position until it gets easier. When this position feels easier, make it harder by:

- Turning your head to the right and to the left
- Looking up

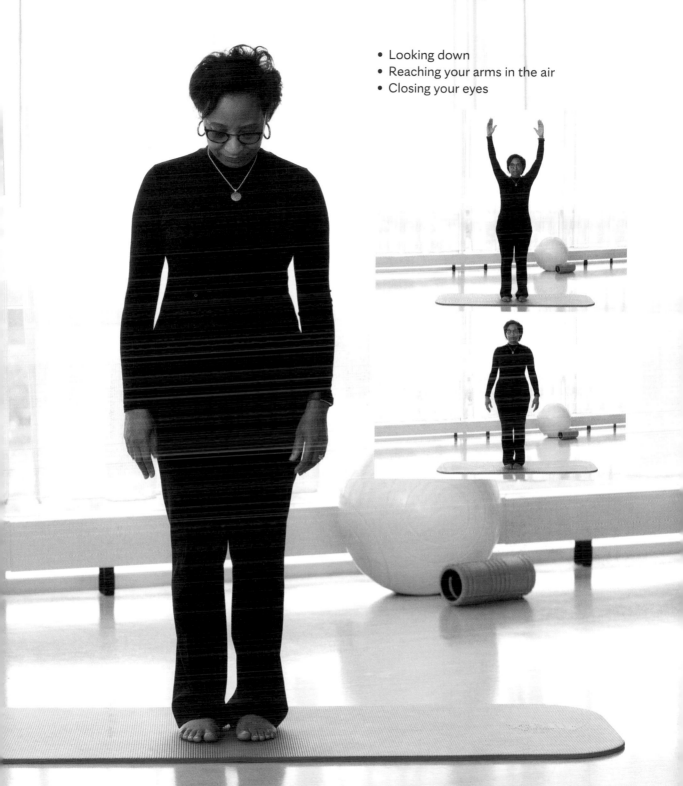

- Looking down
- Reaching your arms in the air
- Closing your eyes

If standing with your feet side by side is easy but you have trouble placing the instep of one foot so that it's touching the big toe of the other foot, practice until you feel comfortable with it. When you're ready to challenge yourself, try:

- Reaching your right arm out while looking to your right
- Reaching your left arm out while looking to your left
- Touching your knees

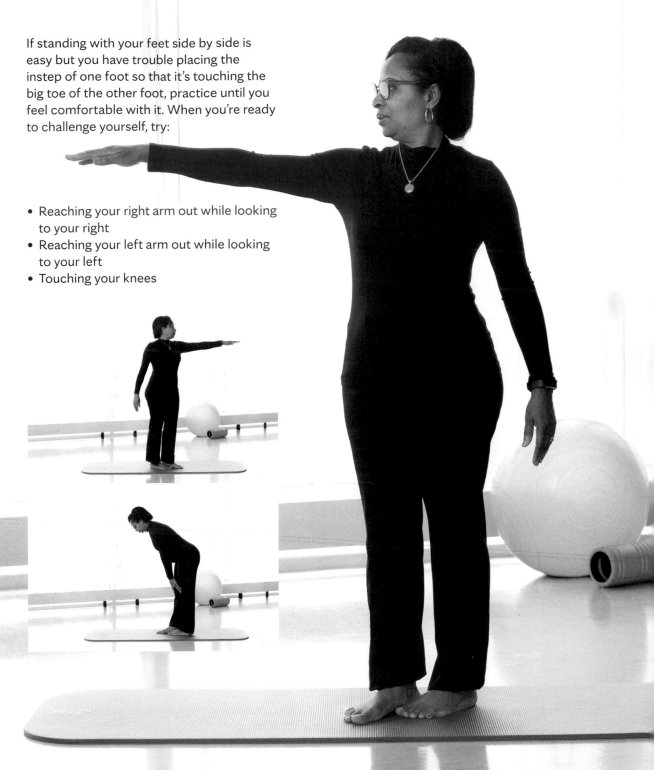

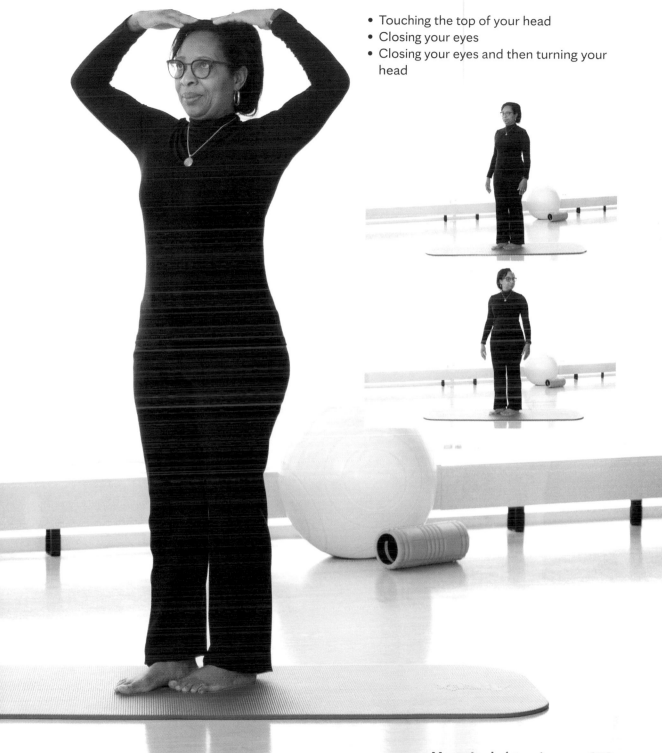

- Touching the top of your head
- Closing your eyes
- Closing your eyes and then turning your head

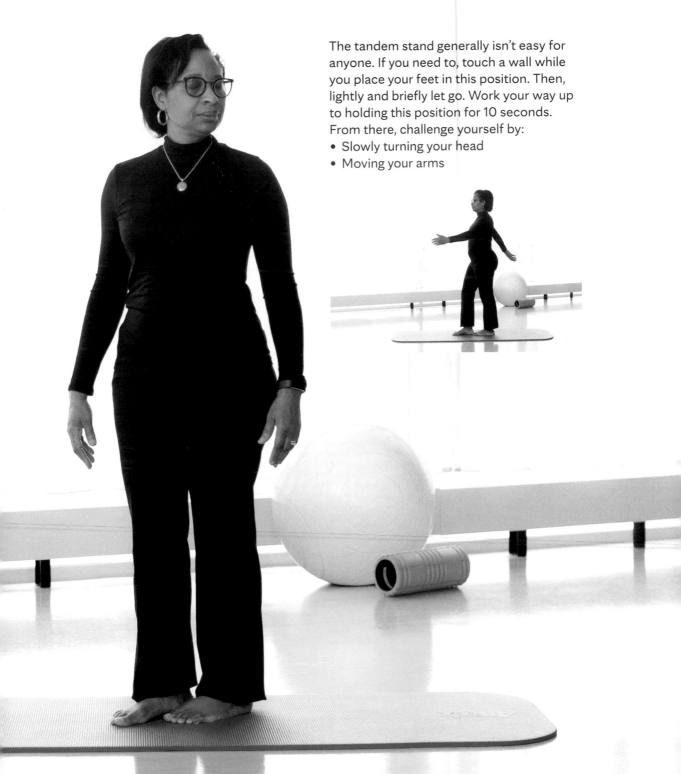

The tandem stand generally isn't easy for anyone. If you need to, touch a wall while you place your feet in this position. Then, lightly and briefly let go. Work your way up to holding this position for 10 seconds. From there, challenge yourself by:

- Slowly turning your head
- Moving your arms

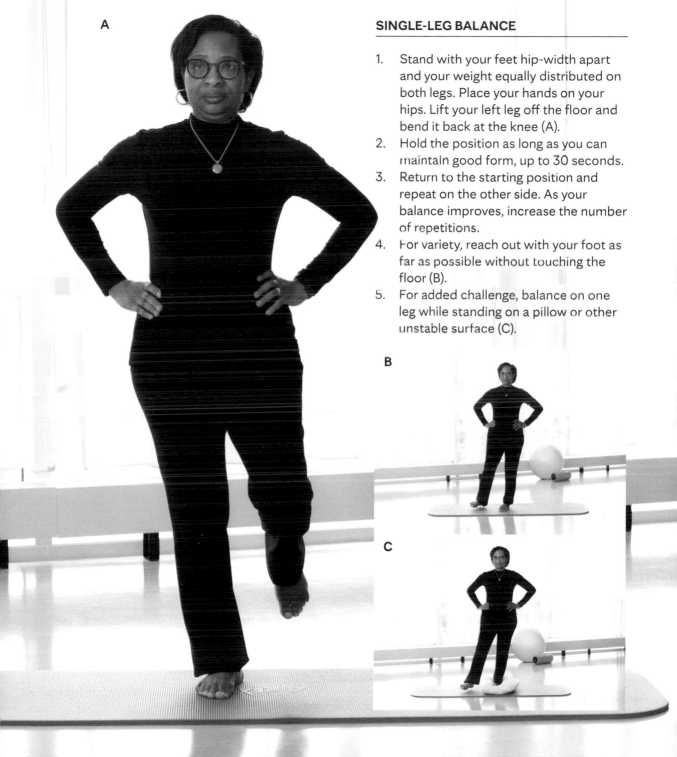

A

SINGLE-LEG BALANCE

1. Stand with your feet hip-width apart and your weight equally distributed on both legs. Place your hands on your hips. Lift your left leg off the floor and bend it back at the knee (A).
2. Hold the position as long as you can maintain good form, up to 30 seconds.
3. Return to the starting position and repeat on the other side. As your balance improves, increase the number of repetitions.
4. For variety, reach out with your foot as far as possible without touching the floor (B).
5. For added challenge, balance on one leg while standing on a pillow or other unstable surface (C).

B

C

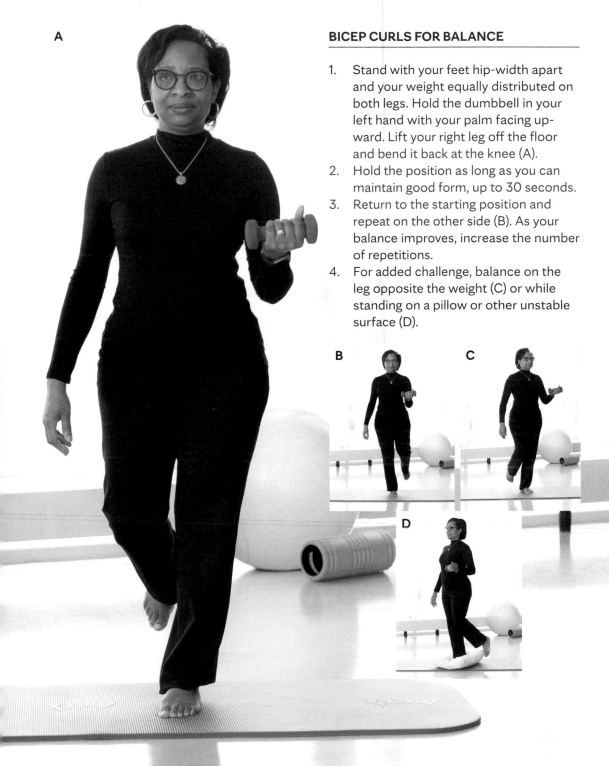

A

BICEP CURLS FOR BALANCE

1. Stand with your feet hip-width apart and your weight equally distributed on both legs. Hold the dumbbell in your left hand with your palm facing upward. Lift your right leg off the floor and bend it back at the knee (A).
2. Hold the position as long as you can maintain good form, up to 30 seconds.
3. Return to the starting position and repeat on the other side (B). As your balance improves, increase the number of repetitions.
4. For added challenge, balance on the leg opposite the weight (C) or while standing on a pillow or other unstable surface (D).

B

C

D

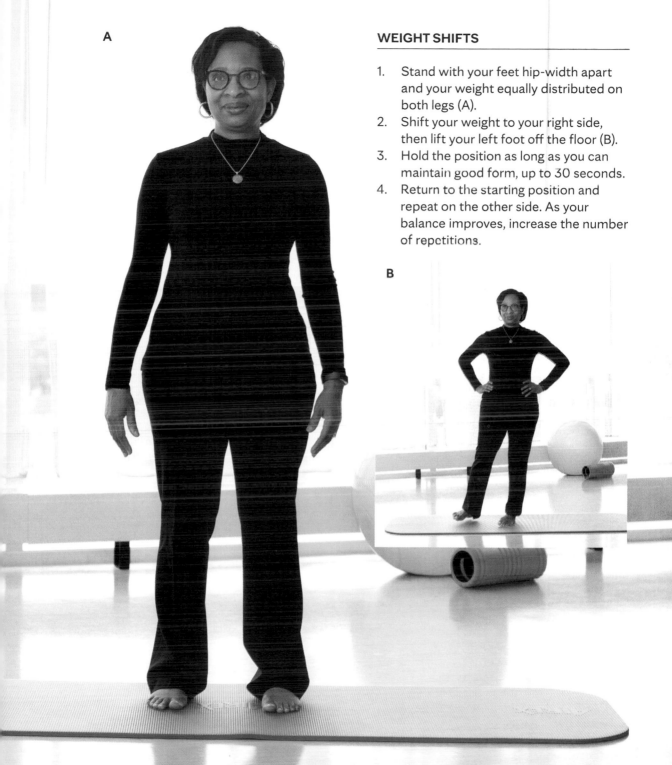

A

WEIGHT SHIFTS

1. Stand with your feet hip-width apart and your weight equally distributed on both legs (A).
2. Shift your weight to your right side, then lift your left foot off the floor (B).
3. Hold the position as long as you can maintain good form, up to 30 seconds.
4. Return to the starting position and repeat on the other side. As your balance improves, increase the number of repetitions.

B

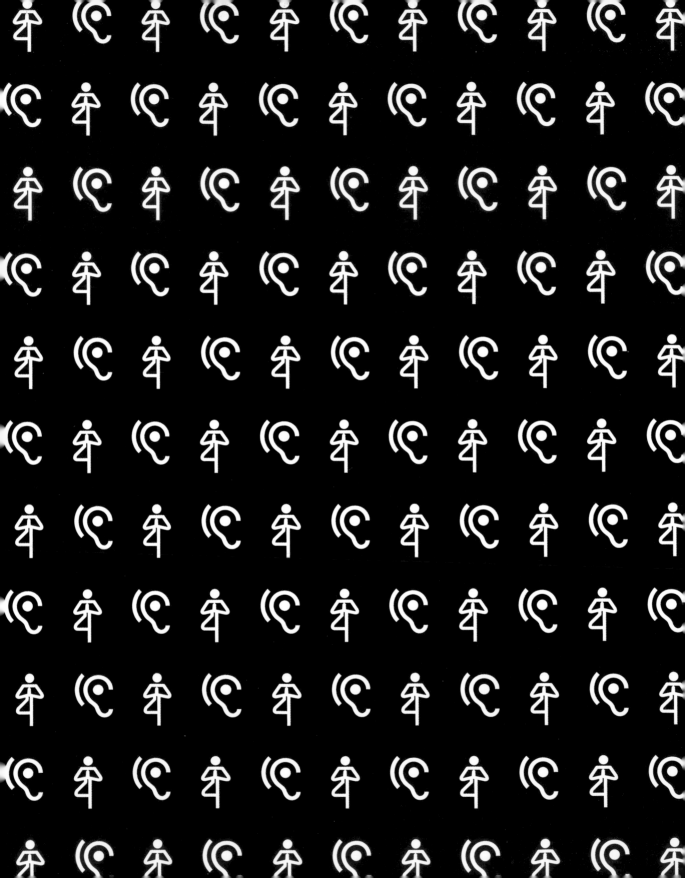

Coping with chronic dizziness

Chronic dizziness has been a part of Joyce's life for most of adulthood. Even in her teens, Joyce experienced clumsiness and a fear of heights — and of falling.

When Joyce stopped taking birth control pills, her dizziness issues became more troublesome. "I began to have increasingly serious bouts of dizziness, always within a day of the onset of each period," Joyce says. "I often had projectile vomiting and had to lie flat, eyes closed, for five hours or more."

As the symptoms continued to worsen, Joyce brought her concerns to her doctor. She was diagnosed with Ménière's disease. Researchers have linked changes in hormone levels to the development of vestibular symptoms, including those of Ménière's disease.

Ultimately, Joyce's doctor prescribed hormone therapy to help prevent dizziness episodes. Hormone therapy and vestibular rehabilitation, which you learned about in Chapter 16, have enabled Joyce to enjoy an active life for nearly four decades. Later in this chapter, you'll get a glimpse into the life Joyce leads today.

CHALLENGES OF CHRONIC DIZZINESS

Chronic dizziness stems from a disorder that affects the balance center in your inner ear or a disorder that affects how balance information is processed by your brain. Your eyes also are affected by dizziness issues; they play a key role in helping you determine where you are in the environment around you.

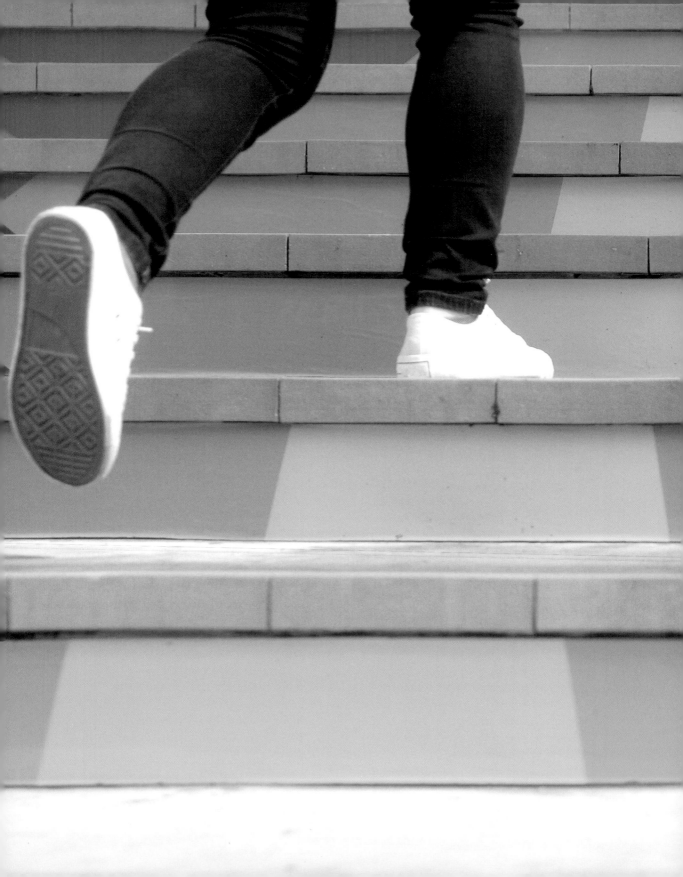

Certain changes in your environment, like pressure changes, movement patterns or lighting, can all cause challenges with chronic dizziness because they affect your ears, your eyes and your sensory system. As a result, chronic dizziness can make it more likely that you'll fall and injure yourself.

Despite the challenges of living with chronic dizziness, you can lessen its effects and enjoy a full and active life. One way is through vestibular rehabilitation, which you learned about earlier. It teaches your eyes, ears and brain ways to adapt to dizziness challenges. With this type of physical therapy, you perform exercises and are gradually exposed to things that make your dizziness worse. The idea is that repeated exposures will help you tolerate and adapt to them. Practiced regularly, vestibular exercises help keep your balance system working well — and help you return to the activities that are important to you.

Along with vestibular rehabilitation, there are many practical ways to keep dizziness episodes to a minimum.

EVERYDAY TIPS

Dizziness occurs when your central nervous system gets information from your eyes that doesn't match up with the information it gets from your ears.

Say you're on an airplane and it experiences turbulence. Your head is likely moving. This triggers the hair cells in your inner ear. Your body is moving, too.

But your eyes don't detect this motion because all you're seeing is the inside of an airplane. As a result, your brain gets mixed messages about what's going on around you, and you may get dizzy or sick.

A similar experience can happen when you're traveling by car. If you're sitting in the back seat reading a book, your inner ear and the rest of your body may be experiencing the bumps and curves along the road, but your eyes are not — they're focused only on the words you're reading. Again, this mismatch of information may cause you to get dizzy or sick.

These are two examples of how miscommunication from one part of your balance system can launch you into a dizziness episode.

Dizziness triggers abound in daily life. They may be so overwhelming that you choose to avoid them at all costs, even if it means missing out on the activities and people you enjoy in life.

In addition to practicing regular vestibular rehabilitation exercises, the following practical tips can help you prevent dizziness episodes and rejoin the people and activities that matter most to you.

Travel

It can be difficult to adjust to the motion you experience during travel — or to the lack of motion after it has stopped. Air travel often includes rapid changes in air pressure that are hard for the ears to regulate. This happens most often when a plane is landing. Likewise, you may experience a similar change in air pressure if you're traveling by train or by car through areas with major elevation changes like mountain passes. And if you travel by train or by boat, you may experience repetitive rocking, swaying or rotating. Bright, dim or flickering light can add to these symptoms. Even people who don't have chronic dizziness often face these challenges.

Although traveling poses challenges for those with chronic dizziness, specific steps can help make traveling manageable and enjoyable. Try these suggestions:

- With your doctor's approval, take a decongestant or nasal spray before you fly on a plane and again before the plane starts to land.
- When your plane is descending, yawn, swallow or chew gum. This helps keep the eustachian tube in your ear open, which helps prevent dizziness issues.
- When booking a hotel room, choose a room on a lower level so that you don't have to use an elevator.
- Choose locations for vacations that don't make your symptoms worse. For example, you may avoid warm or humid climates or destinations that require taking curvy roads.
- On long trips, stop often to get out and walk. This helps your body adjust to the sensation of being on solid ground.
- Avoid reading or working on a computer when traveling by train or car. Instead, focus on what's outside and around you, such as changing scenery. If it's possible, sit in the front seat, facing in the direction you're traveling.

- If you find it tiring or disorienting to stand in long lines or walk through an airport terminal or train station, consider using a cane or holding onto the extended handle of your suitcase.
- Pack items that help with light and sound disturbances. Sunglasses, a hat with a visor, a flashlight and earplugs are all examples.

Dining out

Restaurants can pose challenges for people with chronic dizziness. You may walk into a darkened room, on uneven surfaces, or on carpeting or near walls with complex patterns. A crowded, noisy restaurant with a lot of activity can add to this sensory stimulation. Certain types of light may cause dizziness, lightheadedness, headache and other symptoms related to vestibular disorders.

Keep dizziness triggers to a minimum when dining out by:

- Choosing a restaurant with small, separate rooms
- Avoiding times when there's likely to be a crowd
- Selecting restaurants that don't play loud background music
- Seeking carpeted seating areas that reduce noise and vibrations
- Downloading a menu and choosing your meal before you go so that you don't have to read the menu at the restaurant
- Asking to sit in a corner, away from the kitchen, cash register and bar, so you have fewer people around you
- Choosing a booth instead of a table to help block noise and activity

Attending events

When everything is moving, lighting isn't ideal, and walls aren't nearby for stability, you may struggle to stay balanced. Such is the case at crowded sporting events, in theaters and even walking on city sidewalks with other people. Even simply standing on the sidelines at your child's soccer game may be overwhelming, as you watch the team run back and forth. These situations can be fatiguing for those who struggle with chronic dizziness and balance issues.

To make attending events less taxing, try:
- Using a cane
- Sitting at one end, rather than on the sidelines, when attending a sporting event
- Using a fold-up stool or canvas chair for outdoor events
- Wearing sunglasses and a hat with a brim to calm light and movement

Using screens

Using a computer and watching television can heighten visual sensitivity and make a dizziness episode more likely. While taking breaks from using any kind of screen is good advice, the type of screen you use can go a long way toward preventing visual issues related to dizziness.

Choose a widescreen LCD television and computer monitor. Images are likely to be easier to see and less bright than on other types of screens. Select a computer monitor between 19 and 22 inches, especially if you write and edit documents. This way, you'll be able to scroll less because you can view two full-size pages side by side.

MANAGING STRESS, ANXIETY AND MOOD

Balance disorders can be stressful on many levels. Not knowing when dizziness or vertigo will strike may make you fearful of doing the most basic things, like going to the grocery store or meeting a friend for lunch. And because these disorders aren't visible, perhaps you've been told that your symptoms are imaginary. Just getting a diagnosis can be a lengthy, frustrating process involving many visits to specialists.

So it's not surprising that up to half of the people with balance problems may develop anxiety and depression. These emotional issues can negatively impact balance recovery, leading to symptoms that take longer to resolve. For example, for people with benign paroxysmal positional vertigo (BPPV), researchers have found that treatment is often less helpful for those who also have anxiety and depression.

Anxiety is one of the most common emotional responses linked to balance disorders. Feeling unsteady or having fears of falling can cause people with dizziness or vertigo to avoid social situations or to not leave their homes at all. A vicious cycle begins, with dizziness increasing anxiety and anxiety making dizziness worse. Some people with chronic dizziness also experience panic attacks, adding heart palpitations, sweat-

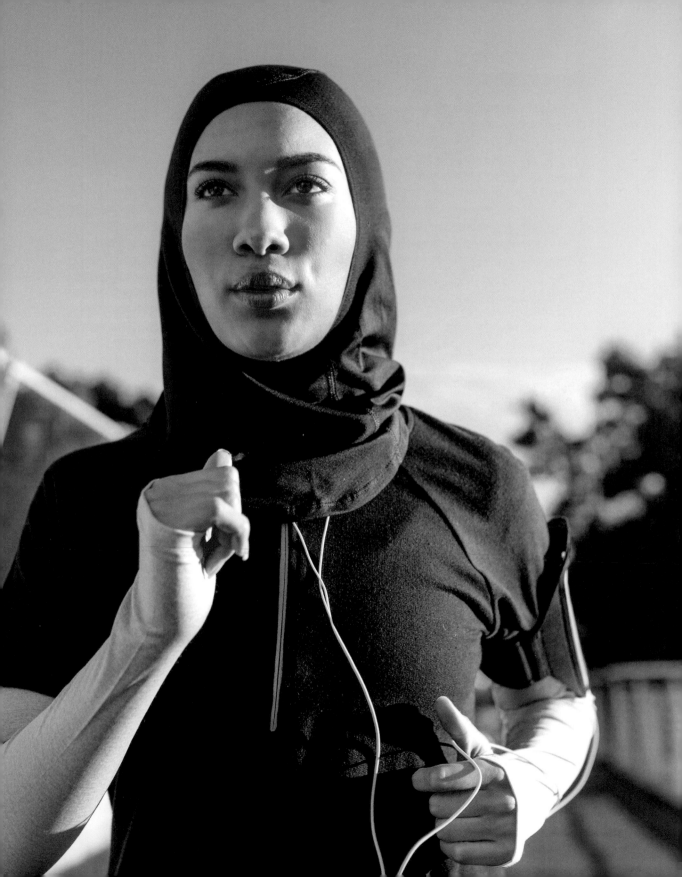

ing, trembling, breathing problems and nausea to the mix.

People with anxiety may wonder if their vestibular problems are a symptom of a mental health condition. That's because sometimes anxiety and depression come first, triggering dizziness. It's important to remember that anxiety stemming from balance issues, no matter which came first, can happen to anyone.

Alongside anxiety, depression can be a side effect of balance issues. Lifestyle changes and loss of independence sometimes caused by balance disorders can make it difficult to enjoy favorite hobbies, go to work or drive a car. These changes can lead to depression. Feeling isolated and misunderstood can make depression worse.

Treating dizziness and its mental health effects

The link between balance and dizziness disorders and stress, anxiety and depression comes down to a basic lesson in how the body and brain are connected. Put simply, anxiety travels along the same nerve pathways that send messages about dizziness to the brain. That's why dizziness and anxiety often go hand in hand. Dizziness tends to increase anxiety, and higher levels of anxiety often lead to feelings of dizziness. This is one more reason to use vestibular rehabilitation to manage chronic dizziness. Vestibular rehabilitation helps train the body and the brain to work together to find new ways to stay balanced.

Cognitive behavioral therapy, along with vestibular rehabilitation, adds the benefit of helping you become aware of inaccurate or negative thinking, so you can view challenging situations more clearly and respond to them in a more effective way.

Cognitive behavioral therapy can be a very helpful tool — either alone or in combination with other therapies — in treating mental health disorders like depression, post-traumatic stress disorder (PTSD) or an eating disorder. It's also especially helpful for those who have anxiety along with dizziness.

Cognitive behavioral therapy can help replace negative thoughts about balance disorders. For example, *I'll never be able to get this dizziness under control!* can be replaced with more-realistic and positive thoughts, such as *I now know what my triggers are, and I'm going to learn how to avoid them.* It also teaches ways to cope with stressful life situations, which can worsen these health problems.

Research suggests that cognitive behavioral therapy, combined with vestibular rehabilitation, reduces dizziness, improves walking, and results in less anxiety and depression in people with persistent dizziness. It can also help identify dizziness triggers, which may help with avoiding anxiety.

Using a therapy that's often part of treatment for mental health conditions doesn't mean that your balance and dizziness issues should be connected to stress or anxiety. But because stress, anxiety and dizziness share the same pathways to the brain, treatment for both dizziness and mental health conditions is helpful.

If you live with chronic dizziness and feel anxious or depressed, take time to recognize when your feelings are caused by your vestibular symptoms. Try keeping a daily journal to keep track of your feelings. You may notice links between your dizziness symptoms and the emotional upheaval you're experiencing. Recognizing this link can help you take steps to manage your feelings when you need to, whether it's through deep breathing, muscle relaxation or guided imagery.

Working with a licensed mental health professional is another step you can take to manage the emotions you're experiencing. Talk with your loved ones about your feelings and enlist their support.

INTEGRATIVE THERAPIES FOR CHRONIC DIZZINESS

Several integrative therapies — also known as complementary or alternative medicine — can help soothe the physical and emotional side effects of chronic dizziness. Here are the therapies that researchers have found help the most.

Mindfulness

Stress is a known trigger for dizziness and vertigo. Moving meditation exercises like yoga, tai chi and Pilates may help improve balance. The exercises can also help with stress management through controlled breathing, relaxation and guided imagery. Yoga, for example, can help quiet the mind and reduce anxiety. Specific yoga poses for balance include the warrior, tree and triangle poses.

When practicing these exercises, you may want to have balance aids — like a chair or wall — nearby.

Biofeedback

Biofeedback helps people adapt to their balance disorders. Movement follows a cycle: An action is started and performed, and any movement errors are detected. A biofeedback device gathers this information about the body, offering a snapshot of how it reacts to a specific movement. Using this information, a person with balance issues can make adjustments to help improve balance.

Various devices offer biofeedback for balance issues. One type features plates that a person stands on, measuring how much a person sways while standing still. Another provides feedback on how balance issues may be affecting a person as he or she walks.

Coaching

Patient education is a key component of managing all aspects of balance issues. As part of a comprehensive treatment plan, it can be helpful to learn all you can about your condition from your health care team, including your abilities and limitations, and whether your balance and dizziness issues are expected to resolve or if you'll need to manage them long term. Your health care team can coach you on how to perform balance improvement tasks and how to adapt or modify movements as needed.

Providers can also educate also provide education about a person's environment — such as the home or work — and what challenges and safety issues may exist in the environment for someone experiencing chronic dizziness. An evaluation of potential home hazards, such as poor lighting and slippery floor surfaces, may be recommended. Modifications such as installing brighter lighting or handrails, placing phones near floor level (in case of a fall), and selecting footwear that's less of a trip or slip hazard may be discussed.

DON'T GIVE UP

At the beginning of this chapter, you learned about Joyce, who's lived with chronic dizziness for most of her life.

At age 78, Joyce leads an active and fulfilling life with Ménière's disease. Nearly 40 years ago, she refused her doctor's initial prescription to quit her job, take Valium and stay in bed. Instead, she's committed herself to the causes and activities she finds most meaningful.

Among them, Joyce has moderated a Ménière's discussion group and has edited, designed, published and distributed books for the Vestibular Disorders Association.

She also regularly volunteers for a program that provides for schoolchildren in need. Every week, she loads 500 loaves — roughly 800 pounds — of donated bread into trucks and then unloads them after driving two hours to a food pantry. "I can still lift 40 pounds shoulder high, which lots of younger people cannot do," Joyce says. Joyce also cuts and hauls wood on the acreage where she lives.

These days, Joyce has noticed that it's more difficult than it used to be for her feet to transmit information to her brain. So, she says, she's learned to listen more carefully.

"The most useful exercise seems to be walking a quarter mile along our gravel road every day, eyes closed for the most part, while concentrating on thinking about what my feet feel," Joyce says.

Joyce's life is a testament to her belief that giving up is never the answer when you encounter a challenge. She encourages people with chronic dizziness to take the steps needed to live life well.

"I believe that all people who have some physical problem can live better if they work at physical therapy or vestibular rehabilitation therapy or whatever it takes to improve their situation — and that it's well worth it!" Joyce says.

Additional resources

Contact these organizations for more information about hearing loss, hearing aids, cochlear implants, and problems with dizziness and imbalance. Some groups offer free publications or videos. Others have publications or videos you can purchase.

Alexander Graham Bell Association for the Deaf and Hard of Hearing
3417 Volta Place NW
Washington, DC 20007
202-337-5220 or 202-337-5221 (TTY)
www.agbell.org

American Academy of Audiology
11480 Commerce Park Drive, Suite 220
Reston, VA 20191
703-790-8466
www.audiology.org

American Academy of Otolaryngology — Head and Neck Surgery
1650 Diagonal Road
Alexandria, VA 22314
703-836-4444
www.entnet.org

American Association of People with Disabilities
2013 H St. NW, Fifth Floor
Washington, DC 20006
202-521-4316 or 800-840-8844 (toll-free)
www.aapd.com

American Auditory Society
P.O. Box 779
Pennsville, NJ 08070
877-746-8315 (toll-free)
www.amauditorysoc.org

American Hearing Research Foundation
275 N. York St., Suite 201
Elmhurst, IL 60126
630-617-5079
www.american-hearing.org

American Society for Deaf Children
P.O. Box 23
Woodbine, MD 21797
800-942-2732 (toll-free)
www.deafchildren.org

American Speech-Language-Hearing Association
2200 Research Blvd.
Rockville, MD 20850-3289
800-638-8255 (toll-free) or
301-296-5650 (TTY)
www.asha.org

American Tinnitus Association
P.O. Box 424049
Washington, DC 20042-4049
800-634-8978 (toll-free)
www.ata.org

Association of Late-Deafened Adults
8038 Macintosh Lane, Suite 2
Rockford, IL 61107-5336
815-332-1515
TTY users, dial 711
www.alda.org

National Association of the Deaf
8630 Fenton St., Suite 820
Silver Spring, MD 20910
301-587-1788 or 301-810-3182 (TTY)
www.nad.org

National Center for Rehabilitative Auditory Research
Portland VA Medical Center
3710 SW U.S. Veterans Hospital Road
P5-NCRAR
Portland, OR 97239
503-220-8262, ext. 55568
www.ncrar.research.va.gov

National Institute on Deafness and Other Communication Disorders
National Institutes of Health
31 Center Drive, MSC 2320
Bethesda, MD 20892-2320
800-241-1044 (toll-free) or
800-241-1055 (TTY)
www.nidcd.nih.gov

Paws With A Cause
4646 Division
Wayland, MI 49348
616-877-7297
www.pawswithacause.org

Vestibular Disorders Association
5018 NE 15th Ave.
Portland, OR 97211
800-837-8428 (toll-free)
www.vestibular.org

Index

M

N

O

P

depression from, 67, 81, 83
describing what you hear, 71
diagnosing, 74
drug therapy for, 75
from earwax blockage, 30
and emotions, 70, 81
and hearing loss, 71
and hyperacusis, 72
integrative therapy for, 78–80, 82
from jaw disorders, 72
masking devices for, 75
from medications, 59, 72
mindfulness meditation for, 80, 82
number of people with, 67
objective (pulsatile), 69–71
from presbycusis, 46
retraining therapy for, 78
from a ruptured eardrum, 33
self-help for, 77
and sleep apnea, 70
and stress, 77, 81
subjective, 71–72, 74
talking to your doctor about, 74
from a tumor, 40
tinnitus treatments
acupuncture, 78–79
biofeedback, 79
cochlear implant, 83
cognitive behavioral therapy, 79–81
deep brain stimulation, 83
diet, 85
health coaching, 80
hearing aids, 75
invasive, 81–84
ketamine, 85
lidocaine, 84
marijuana (cannabis), 84–85
neuromodulation (electrical stimulation), 82
neuromonics, 84
noninvasive, 81–83
transcranial direct stimulation, 82–83

transcranial magnetic stimulation, 82
vagus nerve stimulation, 83–84
tricyclic antidepressants, 75
TRS (Telecommunication Relay Service), 193–194
TRT (tinnitus retraining therapy), 78
tumors
in the ear canal, 33
in the inner ear, 57–59
in the middle ear, 40–41
TV programs with captions, 201–202
tympanomastoidectomy, 39

U

Usher's syndrome type 3, 55

V

vagus nerve stimulation, 83–84
VEMP (vestibular evoked myogenic potential) test, 225
vertigo
with alcohol use, 60, 229
causes of, 247
after cochlear implant surgery, 181
common causes of, 229
with labyrinthitis, 57
with Ménière's disease, 55
from third window disorders, 231
with vestibular disorders, 217
when to be concerned about, 222
See also balance problems/disorders; balance problems/disorders, managing; BPPV; dizziness
vestibular labyrinth
defined, 15
and dizziness, 217
how it helps you balance, 19, 22, 24, 218–219
vestibular migraine, 229–230
vestibular neuritis, 56–57

W

X

Y

Image credits

The individuals pictured are models, and the photos are used for illustrative purposes only. There's no correlation between the individuals portrayed and the condition or subject discussed. All photographs and illustrations are copyright of MFMER except for the following: NAME: shutterstock_567939001/PAGE: Cover/CREDIT: © SHUTTERSTOCK NAME: shutterstock_477963706.jpg/ PAGE: 20/CREDIT: © SHUTTERSTOCK NAME: shutterstock_231222595.jpg/PAGE: 23/CREDIT: © SHUTTERSTOCK NAME: shutterstock_411246616.jpg/ PAGE: 24/CREDIT: © SHUTTERSTOCK NAME: shutterstock_678902572.jpg/PAGE: 76/CREDIT: © SHUTTERSTOCK NAME: shutterstock_1893768634. jpg/PAGE: 77/CREDIT: © SHUTTERSTOCK. NAME: shutterstock_238671202.jpg/PAGE: 80/ CREDIT: © SHUTTERSTOCK. NAME: shutterstock_755581873.jpg/ PAGE: 126/ CREDIT: © SHUTTERSTOCK. NAME: shutterstock_1177754176.jpg/PAGE: 138/ CREDIT: © SHUTTERSTOCK. NAME: shutterstock_1285054693. jpg/PAGE: 155/ CREDIT: © SHUTTERSTOCK. NAME: shutterstock_157378409.jpg/PAGE: 166/ CREDIT: © SHUTTERSTOCK. NAME: shutterstock_1349505794. jpg/PAGE: 232/ CREDIT: © SHUTTERSTOCK. NAME: GettyImages-1291312257.jpg/PAGE: 249/ CREDIT: © Getty. NAME: shutterstock_723086374.jpg/PAGE: 264/ CREDIT: © SHUTTERSTOCK. NAME: shutterstock_723086374.jpg/PAGE: 266/ CREDIT: © SHUTTERSTOCK. NAME: shutterstock_1247806225. jpg/PAGE: 268/ CREDIT: © SHUTTERSTOCK. NAME: sshutterstock_1247806225.jpg/PAGE: 270/ CREDIT: © SHUTTERSTOCK.

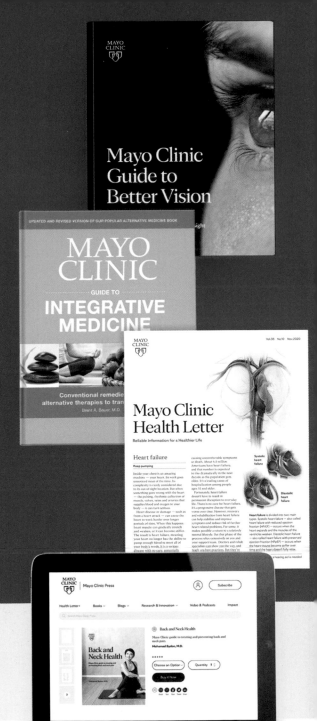